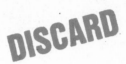

PHARMACY TECHNICIAN EXAM

Related Titles

Becoming a Healthcare Professional
Health Occupations Entrance Exams

PHARMACY TECHNICIAN EXAM

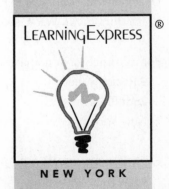

NEW YORK

Pharmacy technician exam.
    p.; cm.
  ISBN-13: 978-1-57685-737-3
  ISBN-10: 1-57685-737-9
 1. Pharmacy technicians—Examinations, questions, etc. I.
LearningExpress (Organization)
  [DNLM: 1. Pharmacy—Examination Questions. 2. Pharmacists' Aides.
QV 18.2 P5369 2010]
  RS122.95.P44 2010
  615'.1076—dc22

                                                    2010012751

Printed in the United States of America

9 8 7 6 5 4 3 2

ISBN-13: 978-1-57685-737-3

Developed and illustrated by Focus Strategic Communications, Inc.
Project Managers: Ron Edwards, Adrianna Edwards
Development Editors: Ron Edwards, Jenna Dunlop
Illustrators: Sarah Waterfield, Carolyn Tripp

For information or to place an order, contact LearningExpress at:
  2 Rector Street
  26th Floor
  New York, NY 1,0006

Or visit us at:
  www.learnatest.com

CONTENTS

CONTRIBUTORS ▶

Thomas Fridley, CPhT, is pursuing his doctor of pharmacy degree at Long Island University. He received his certification in 2004 from the pharmacy technician Certification Board. During his practice years, he was a pharmacy technician for Eckerd pharmacy and the Regional Intern Program Manager for CVS. Currently, he is the pharmacy Technology Program Chair at the Sanford-Brown Institute in Garden City—the first school in New York State to receive American Society of Health System Pharmacists accreditation for its technician program.

Joe Medina, CPhT, BS, is the former program director of two ASHP-accredited pharmacy technician programs at two community colleges in Colorado. He has worked in retail, in-patient hospital and state psychiatric hospital pharmacy settings, and is well known as a national advocate for the pharmacy technician profession. Medina helped produce several textbooks and coauthored the *Pharmacy Technician Workbook & Certification Review* through Morton Publishing. With 15 years as a pharmacy technician and 20 years as a pharmacist, Medina is an advocate for the needs of pharmacy technicians and the important role they play for pharmacists, medical paraprofessionals, and the pharmacy community.

Michael Spencer, BA, PharmD, graduated from the University of California, Berkeley, with a degree in biochemistry and the University of California, San Francisco, with a doctor of pharmacy degree. He has four decades of pharmacy practice experience in community, hospital, and research facilities and over two decades of experience teaching both pharmacists and pharmacy technicians. He is currently Director of pharmacy Services at Memorial Medical Center in Modesto, CA, and Program Director for the pharmacy technician Career Training Program at Modesto Junior College.

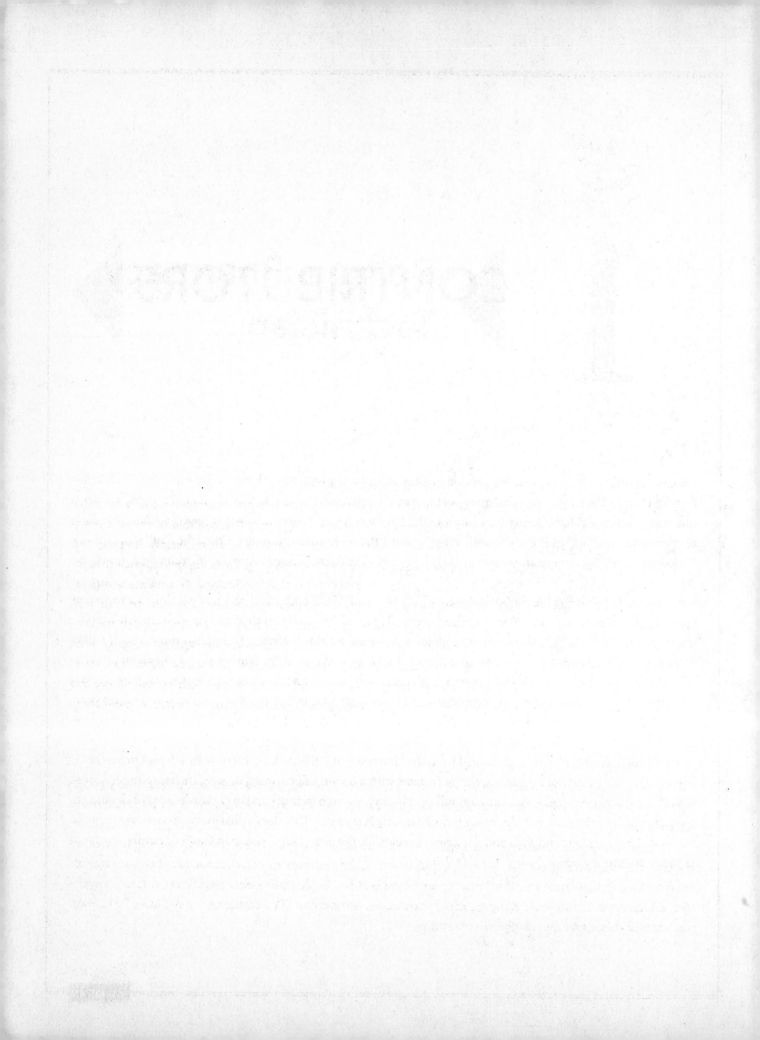

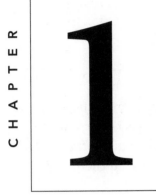

Being a Pharmacy Technician

CHAPTER OVERVIEW

Although the pharmacy technician profession has been around for many years, it was not until recently that the role of the pharmacy technician has changed dramatically, from simply helping the pharmacist in the pharmacy setting to actually dispensing functions in the filling of prescription/medication/IV admixture orders. In the past, many pharmacy technicians learned on the job, trained by the pharmacists, but today we are finding that responsibility has increased for pharmacy technicians, along with accountability. With this in mind, the pharmacy technician vocation is facing a change, with national certification becoming the norm in most states, as well as state-based registration and licensing for individual pharmacy technicians.

B eing a pharmacy technician offers an exciting opportunity to help others in the healthcare setting as one who not only assists the pharmacist, but also plays a vital role in dispensing prescription/medication orders.

Opportunities for advancement are many, as the individual pharmacy technician may see employment in not only the retail setting, but the hospital setting as well. Other avenues of specialization for pharmacy technicians include (but are not limited to) mail order, home healthcare, pharmaceutical companies, insurance agencies, educational institutions, compounding pharmacies, intravenous (IV) admixture preparation, and both nuclear and chemotherapeutic pharmacy settings.

The role of the pharmacy technician has changed from working the cash register to actually filling prescriptions and medication orders. Today, 95% of these orders are filled by pharmacy technicians. With this in mind, the need for national standardization has become a concern to ensure pharmacy technicians have the educational background to perform these functions. Although most states do not require formal education, states are beginning to recognize the importance of national certification.

Functions of pharmacy technicians vary according to which pharmacy setting they work in, and the duties the pharmacist allows them to do. Most functions involve filling prescriptions (retail setting) or filling medication orders and making IV admixtures (both hospital settings).

In the retail pharmacy, the pharmacy technician may receive a written prescription from a patient, enter information into the computer, and fill the prescription order. Any task requiring a judgment or decision is performed by the pharmacist. This would include taking new prescription orders, making a final check of a filled prescription order, and counseling patients.

In the hospital setting, the filling of medication orders is done in individual patient units we call a *cassette tray*, filled with individual prepackaged units of medication(s) called *unit doses*. This is done by the pharmacy technician as well, although medication orders are generally entered by the pharmacist to ensure accuracy and identify potential problems (such as drug interactions and the like). The hospital setting also offers the pharmacy technician the opportunity to make IV admixtures and chemotherapeutic IV drugs. Again, all roles requiring a judgmental decision are performed by the pharmacist, such as the final check of a medication/IV admixture order or clinical discussions with hospital staff.

All of these disciplines will be discussed in later chapters.

Education and Certification

As mentioned earlier, most states are now requiring their pharmacy technicians to be nationally certified. Currently, there are two regulatory national organizations that offer national certification; they are the pharmacy technician Certification Board (PTCB), which offers the pharmacy technician Certification Exam (PTCE); and the Institute for the Certification of pharmacy technicians (ICPT), which offers the Exam for the Certification of pharmacy technicians (ExCPT). Check the requirements of your state and your employer to determine which regulatory organization you would choose for your national certification.

Passing either national exam does certify the pharmacy technician, and allows him or her to wear the letters CPhT (Certified pharmacy technician). This tells the consumer that the pharmacy technician has passed a valid national exam and has displayed competency in his or her duties in the pharmacy.

The PTCB exam consists of 90 multiple-choice questions and is offered in the computer format to be taken on demand or when scheduled. The time limit is 110 minutes. The ExCPT exam consists of 110 multiple-choice questions. The time limit is 120 minutes. Both exams have ten experimental questions which do not count against the overall score, which the test makers evaluate to see if they should be used in future exams. A pass/fail notice is given upon completion of each exam. For specific information on each exam, go to the following links:

PTCB: www.ptcb.org
ICPT: www.nationaltechexam.org

Only a handful of states mandate receiving a specific state certificate of completion in an accredited pharmacy technician program, including Ohio and Florida. For now, it appears the national exams are the standard as far as accountability for the pharmacy technician. For specifics of what your state requires, you need to check with your state board of pharmacy, as changes do occur rapidly in this field.

National Association of Boards of pharmacy or NABP: www.nabp.net/boards-of-pharmacy

Certification requires pharmacy technicians to complete 20 hours of continuing education (CE) every two years to maintain their national certification. Continuing education shows that the pharmacy technician is keeping up with what is new in the pharmacy industry. CE is offered by a number of sources, including Internet sites which offer pharmacy technician–specific CE, colleges, pharmacy employers, pharmacy magazines, journals, or associations, to name some. One such organization that has been around for more than 14 years is Tech Lectures, which offers affordable pharmacy technician–specific CE. Another company is PowerPak, which offers CE for free. Just realize that CE should be about learning to enhance both personal and professional growth, and not just getting those required recertification hours.

Tech Lectures: www.tlectures.com
PowerPak: www.powerpak.com

Economic Outlook

Today, the pharmacy technician field is growing at a rapid rate, with a projected growth rate of 25% until the year 2013—with a 31% increase, according to the United States Bureau of Labor and Statistics (USBLS).

Pharmacy technician wages differ from state to state and employer to employer. In many cases, it is dependent on supply versus demand and the type of pharmacy where the pharmacy technician works. Generally, the more specialized pharmacy setting the pharmacy technician works in, the higher the wages earned. According to the USBLS May 2009 National Occupational Employment and Wage Estimates, mean wages range from $9.36 per hour (or approximately $19,480 per year) up to $19.31 per hour (or

approximately $40,160 per year). Wages may also be higher or lower than the national means, depending on factors like the ones mentioned above. The USBLS estimates that there are currently 331,900 pharmacy technicians.

Pharmacy Technician Associations

Once you are a pharmacy technician, it is important that you try to join a professional association, whether it's a pharmacists' association that has a specific pharmacy technician unit, or a national organization that is specifically for and about pharmacy technicians. These associations help in networking with fellow pharmacy technicians, developing friendships with others in your vocation, and finding job opportunities.

The American Association of pharmacy technicians (AAPT) (www.pharmacytechnician.com) was established in 1979 and is currently the organization of choice for many pharmacy technicians, due to its longevity and how it caters to its membership base. The organization offers CE, as well as one yearly national convention and seminars throughout the year in different states. The American Association of Pharmacy Technicians is run by volunteers and has state chapters which you may join—or decide to start your own!

Be wary, though, when selecting an organization (or several) to belong to, as there are organizations that seem more interested in your membership dues than in really serving your individual needs. You have a choice in what serves your better interest, as there are many out there who will gladly take your money but offer little.

Time to Begin

The pharmacy technician field is an exciting career avenue for one interested in helping those in need, whether it's in a retail, hospital, or specialized setting. You work side by side with fellow technicians and other health professionals to not only enhance the quality of lives of customers/patients you serve, but in some cases, to save lives as well. In this vocation, you are given the opportunity to continue to learn as you develop your skills and pursue/advance to other pharmacy settings. For some, this is will be your vocation for life—and for others, this may be a stepping stone to another health profession, as some continue onward to get their doctor of pharmacy degree and become full pharmacists.

With this in mind, you have decided to pursue becoming a pharmacy technician; and you have most likely purchased this review book to learn as much as you can to help you pass one of the national exams. This book will allow you that opportunity, but you must put effort into the learning process. That is your first step on your way to being recognized as a nationally certified pharmacy technician!

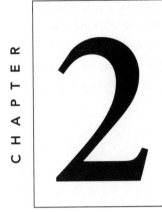

The LearningExpress Test Preparation System

CHAPTER OVERVIEW

Taking any written exam can be tough. It demands a lot of preparation if you want to achieve a top score. Your rank on the eligibility list is often determined largely by this score. The LearningExpress Test Preparation System, developed exclusively for LearningExpress by leading test experts, gives you the discipline and attitude you need to be a winner.

Taking this written exam is no picnic, and neither is getting ready for it. Your future career in pharmacy technology depends on you getting a high score on the various parts of the test, but there are all sorts of pitfalls that can keep you from doing your best on this all-important exam. Here are some of the obstacles that can stand in the way of your success:

- being unfamiliar with the format of the exam
- being paralyzed by test anxiety
- leaving your preparation to the last minute or not preparing at all
- not knowing vital test-taking skills—how to pace yourself through the exam, how to use the process of elimination, and when to guess
- not being in tip-top mental and physical shape
- messing up on test day by having to work on an empty stomach or shivering through the exam because the room is cold

What's the common denominator in all these test-taking pitfalls? One word: control. Who's in control, you or the exam?

Now the good news: The LearningExpress Test Preparation System puts you in control. In just nine easy-to-follow steps, you will learn everything you need to know to make sure that you are in charge of your preparation and your performance on the exam. Other test takers may let the test get the better of them; they may be unprepared or out of shape, but not you. You will have taken all the steps you need to take to get a high score on the pharmacy technician exam.

Here's how the LearningExpress Test Preparation System works: Nine easy steps lead you through everything you need to know and do to get ready to master your exam. Each of the steps listed below includes both reading about the step and one or more activities. It's important that you do the activities along with the reading, or you won't be getting the full benefit of the system. Each step tells you approximately how much time it will take to complete.

Step 1: Get Information   (30 minutes)
Step 2: Conquer Test Anxiety   (20 minutes)
Step 3: Make a Plan   (50 minutes)
Step 4: Learn to Manage Your Time   (10 minutes)
Step 5: Learn to Use the Process of Elimination   (20 minutes)
Step 6: Know When to Guess   (20 minutes)
Step 7: Reach Your Peak Performance Zone   (10 minutes)
Step 8: Get Your Act Together   (10 minutes)
Step 9: Do It!   (10 minutes)

Total time for complete system (180 minutes—3 hours)

We estimate that working through the entire system will take you approximately three hours, though it's perfectly okay if you work faster or slower. If you can take a whole afternoon or evening, you can work through the whole LearningExpress Test Preparation System in one sitting. Otherwise, you can break it up, and do just one or two steps a day for the next several days. It's up to you—remember, you're in control.

Step 1: Get Information

Time to complete: 30 minutes
Activities: Read Introduction, "How to Use this Book"
Knowledge is power. The first step in the LearningExpress Test Preparation System is finding out everything you can about the pharmacy technician exams offered. For example, the PTCB or ICPT website outlines all the details about taking their national exams. Your state board of pharmacy will have information for you concerning their own requirements for being a pharmacy technician and what exams need to be taken, which varies from state to state.

What You Should Find Out
The more details you can find out about the exam, either from the national or state board's publications, the more efficiently you will be able to study. Here's a list of some things you will want to find out about your exam:

- What skills are tested?
- How many sections are on the exam?
- How many questions are in each section?
- Are the questions ordered from easy to hard, or is the sequence random?
- How much time is allotted for each section?
- Are there breaks between sections?
- What is the passing score, and how many questions do you have to answer correctly in order to pass?
- How is the test scored? Is there a penalty for wrong answers?
- Are you permitted to go back to a prior section or move on to the next section if you finish early?
- Can you write in the test booklet, or will you be given scratch paper?
- What should you bring with you on exam day?

What's on Most Pharmacy Technician Exams

The skills that are tested on either of the pharmacy technician national exams are standardized.

If you haven't already done so, stop here and read Chapter 1 of this book, which gives you an overview of the entire process of becoming a pharmacy technician. Then move on to the next step and get rid of that test anxiety.

Step 2: Conquer Test Anxiety

Time to complete: 20 minutes

Activity: Take the Test Anxiety Quiz (page 9)

Having complete information about the test is the first step in getting control of the exam. Next, you have to overcome one of the biggest obstacles to test success: test anxiety. Test anxiety can not only impair your performance on the exam itself, it can even keep you from preparing properly. In Step 2, you will learn stress management techniques that will help you succeed on your exam. Learn these strategies now, and practice them as you work through the questions in this book, so they'll be second nature to you by exam day.

Combating Test Anxiety

The first thing you need to know is that a little test anxiety is a good thing. Everyone gets nervous before a big exam—and if that nervousness motivates you to prepare thoroughly, so much the better. It's said that Sir Laurence Olivier, one of the foremost British actors of the twentieth century, threw up before every performance. His stage fright didn't impair his performance; in fact, it probably gave him a little extra edge—just the kind of edge you need to do well, whether on a stage or in an examination room.

On page 9 is the Test Anxiety Quiz. Stop here and answer the questions on that page, to find out whether your level of test anxiety is something you should worry about.

Stress Management Before the Test

If you feel your level of anxiety is getting the best of you in the weeks before the test, here is what you need to do to bring the level down again:

- **Get prepared.** There's nothing like knowing what to expect and being prepared for it to put you in control of test anxiety. That's why you're reading this book. Use it faithfully, and remind yourself that you're better prepared than most of the people taking the test.

- **Practice self-confidence.** A positive attitude is a great way to combat test anxiety. This is no time to be humble or shy. Stand in front of the mirror and say to your reflection, "I'm prepared. I'm full of self-confidence. I'm going to ace this test. I know I can do it." Record it on an iPod or MP3 player and play it back once a day. If you hear it often enough, you will believe it.

- **Fight negative messages.** Every time someone starts telling you how hard the exam is or how it's almost impossible to get a high score, start repeating your self-confidence messages above. If the person with the negative messages is you—telling yourself you don't do well on exams, that you just can't do this—don't listen. Turn on your iPod and listen to your self-confidence messages.

- **Visualize.** Imagine yourself reporting for duty on your first day of pharmacy technology training. Think of yourself wearing your uniform with pride and learning skills you will use for the rest of your life. Visualizing success can help make it happen—and it reminds you why you're doing all this work preparing for the exam.

- **Exercise.** Physical activity helps calm your body and focus your mind. Besides, being in good physical shape can actually help you do well on the exam. Go for a run, lift weights, go swimming—and do it regularly.

Stress Management on Test Day

There are several ways you can bring down your level of test stress and anxiety on test day. They'll work best if you practice them in the weeks before the test so you know which ones work best for you.

- **Deep breathing.** Take a deep breath while you count to five. Hold it for a count of one, and then let it out on a count of five. Repeat several times.

- **Move your body.** Try rolling your head in a circle. Rotate your shoulders. Shake your hands from the wrist. Many people find these movements very relaxing.

- **Visualize again.** Think of the place where you are most relaxed: lying on the beach in the sun, walking through the park, or whatever. Now, close your eyes and imagine you're actually there. If you practice in advance, you will find that you only need a few seconds of this exercise to experience a significant increase in your sense of well-being.

When anxiety threatens to overwhelm you *during the exam*, there are still things you can do to manage the stress level:

- **Repeat your self-confidence messages.** You should have them memorized by now. Say them quietly to yourself, and believe them!

- **Visualize one more time.** This time, visualize yourself moving smoothly and quickly through the test, answering every question right and finishing just before time is up. Like most visualization techniques, this one works best if you've practiced ahead of time.

- **Find an easy question.** Skim over the test until you find an easy question, and answer it. Getting even one circle filled in gets you into the test-taking groove.

Test Anxiety Quiz

You need to worry about test anxiety only if it is extreme enough to impair your performance. The following questionnaire will provide a diagnosis of your level of test anxiety. In the blank before each statement, write the number that most accurately describes your experience.

0 = Never
1 = Once or twice
2 = Sometimes
3 = Often

___ I have gotten so nervous before an exam that I simply put down the books and didn't study for it.

___ I have experienced disabling physical symptoms such as vomiting and severe headaches because I was nervous about an exam.

___ I have simply not showed up for an exam because I was scared to take it.

___ I have experienced dizziness and disorientation while taking an exam.

___ I have failed an exam because I was too nervous to complete it.

___ **Total (Add up the numbers in the blanks above.)**

Your Test Stress Score

Here are the steps you should take, depending on your score. If you scored:

- **Below 3:** Your level of test anxiety is nothing to worry about; it's probably just enough to give you that little extra edge.
- **Between 3 and 6:** Your test anxiety may be enough to impair your performance, and you should practice the stress management techniques listed in this section to try to bring your test anxiety down to manageable levels.
- **Above 6:** Your level of test anxiety is a serious concern. In addition to practicing the stress management techniques listed in this section, you may want to seek additional, personal help. Call your local high school or community college and ask for the academic counselor. Tell the counselor that you have a level of test anxiety that sometimes keeps you from being able to take the exam. The counselor may be willing to help you or may suggest someone else you should talk to.

- **Take a mental break.** Everyone loses concentration once in a while during a long test. It's normal, so you shouldn't worry about it. Instead, accept what has happened. Say to yourself, "Hey, I lost it there for a minute. My brain is taking a break." Put down your pencil, close your eyes, and do some deep breathing for a few seconds. Then you're ready to go back to work.

Try these techniques ahead of time, and see if they work for you!

Step 3: Make a Plan

Time to complete: 50 minutes
Activity: Construct a study plan
Maybe the most important thing you can do to get control of yourself and your exam is to make a study plan. Too many people fail to prepare simply because they fail to plan. Spending hours on the day before the exam poring over sample test questions not only raises your level of test anxiety, it is no substitute for careful preparation and practice over time.

Don't fall into the cram trap. Take control of your preparation time by mapping out a study schedule. There are four sample schedules on the following pages, based on the amount of time you have before the exam. If you're the kind of person who needs deadlines and assignments to motivate you for a project, here they are. If you're the kind of person who doesn't like to follow other people's plans, you can use the suggested schedules to construct your own.

In constructing your plan, you should take into account how much work you need to do. If your score on the sample test wasn't what you had hoped, consider taking some of the steps from Schedule A and fitting them into Schedule D, even if you do have only three weeks before the exam. **You can also customize your plan according to the information you gathered in Step 1.**

Even more important than making a plan is making a commitment. You can't improve your skills in reading, writing, and judgment overnight. You have to set aside some time every day for study and practice. Try for at least 20 minutes a day. Twenty minutes daily will do you much more good than two hours crammed into a Saturday.

If you have months before the exam, you're lucky. Don't put off your study until the week before the exam! Start now. Even ten minutes a day, with half an hour or more on weekends, can make a big difference in your score.

Schedule A: The Leisure Plan

This schedule gives you six months to sharpen your skills. If an exam is announced in the middle of your preparation, you can use one of the later schedules to help you compress your study program. Only study the chapters that are relevant to the type of exam you will be taking.

TIME	PREPARATION
Exam minus six months	Answer the questions from Chapter 3: diagnostic test. Then study the explanations for the answers until you know you could answer all the questions correctly.
Exam minus five months	Read Chapters 4 and 5 and work through the exercises. Use at least one of the additional resources for each chapter. Start going to the library once every two weeks to read books or magazines about pharmacy. Find other people who are preparing for the test and form a study group.
Exam minus four months	Read Chapters 6, 7, and 8 and work through the exercises. Use at least one of the additional resources for each chapter. Remember to read up on pharmacy math and to go over your top 100 drug list.
Exam minus three months	Read Chapters 9, 10, and 11 and work through the exercises. Use at least one of the additional resources for each chapter. Locate other pharmacy calculation type problems to better your individual skills. Remember to go over your top 100 drug list.
Exam minus two months	Read Chapter 12 and work through the exercises. Continue practicing your pharmacy calculation problems and memorizing your top 100 drug list.
Exam minus one month	Take the practice test in Chapter 13. Use your score to help you decide where to concentrate your efforts this month. Go back to the relevant chapters and use the additional resources listed there, or get the help of a friend or teacher. Repeat the whole process with the first and second online tests.
Exam minus one week	Review the sample questions. See how much you've learned in the past months. Concentrate on what you've done well, and decide not to let any areas where you still feel uncertain bother you.
Exam minus one day	Relax. Do something unrelated to the pharmacy technician exams. Eat a good meal and go to bed at your usual time.

SCHEDULE B: THE JUST-ENOUGH-TIME PLAN

If you have three to six months before the exam, that should be enough time to prepare for the written test, especially if you score above 70 on the first sample test you take. This schedule assumes four months; stretch it out or compress it if you have more or less time, and only study the chapters that are relevant to the type of exam you will be taking.

TIME	PREPARATION
Exam minus four months	Take the diagnostic test in Chapter 3 to determine where you need the most work. Read Chapters 4 through 8 and work through the exercises. Use at least one of the additional resources listed in each chapter. Start going to the library once every two weeks to read books about pharmacy technician topics.
Exam minus three months	Read Chapters 9, 10, and 11 and work through the exercises.
Exam minus two months	Read Chapter 12, and work through the exercises. You're still doing your reading, aren't you?
Exam minus one month	Take the practice test in Chapter 13. Use your score to help you decide where to concentrate your efforts this month. Go back to the relevant chapters and use the additional resources listed there, or get the help of a friend or teacher. Repeat the whole process with the first and second online tests.
Exam minus one week	Review the sample questions. See how much you've learned in the past months. Concentrate on what you've done well, and decide not to let any areas where you still feel uncertain bother you.
Exam minus one day	Relax. Do something unrelated to pharmacy technician exams. Eat a good meal and go to bed at your usual time.

Schedule C: More Study in Less Time

If you have one to three months before the exam, you still have enough time for some concentrated study that will help you improve your score. This schedule is built around a two-month time frame. If you have only one month, spend an extra couple of hours a week to get all these steps in. If you have three months, take some of the steps from Schedule B and fit them in. Only study the chapters that are relevant to the type of exam you will be taking.

TIME	PREPARATION
Exam minus eight weeks	Take the sample diagnostic test in Chapter 3 to find one or two areas you're weakest in. Choose the appropriate chapter(s) from among Chapters 4–13 to read in these first two weeks. Use some of the additional resources listed there.
Exam minus six weeks	Read Chapters 4–8 and work through the exercises.
Exam minus four weeks	Read Chapters 9–12 and work through the exercises.
Exam minus two weeks	Take the practice test in Chapter 13. Use your score to help you decide where to concentrate your efforts this month. Go back to the relevant chapters and use the additional resources listed there, or get the help of a friend or teacher. Repeat the whole process with the first and second online tests.
Exam minus one week	Review the sample questions, concentrating on the areas where a little work can help the most.

TIME	PREPARATION
Exam minus one day	Relax. Do something unrelated to pharmacy technician exams. Eat a good meal and go to bed at your usual time.

Schedule D: The Cram Plan

If you have three weeks or less before the exam, you really have your work cut out for you. Carve half an hour out of your day, every day, for study. This schedule assumes you have the whole three weeks to prepare; if you have less time, you will have to compress the schedule accordingly. Only study the chapters that are relevant to the type of exam you will be taking.

TIME	PREPARATION
Exam minus three weeks	Take the diagnostic test in Chapter 3. Then read the material in Chapters 4–8 and work through the exercises.
Exam minus two weeks	Read the material in Chapters 9–12 and work through the exercises. Take the Chapter 13 practice test followed by a sample online test, score them, and review your areas of weakness.
Exam minus one week	Evaluate your performance on the second online sample test. Review the parts of Chapters 4–12 that you had the most trouble with. Get a friend or teacher to help you with the section you had the most difficulty with.
Exam minus two days	Review the diagnostic test in Chapter 3, the Chapter 13 practice test, and the two online tests. Make sure you understand the answer explanations.
Exam minus one day	Relax. Do something unrelated to pharmacy technician exams. Eat a good meal and go to bed at your usual time.

Step 4: Learn to Manage Your Time

Time to complete: 10 minutes to read, many hours of practice
Activities: Practice these strategies as you take the sample tests in this book

Steps 4, 5, and 6 of the LearningExpress Test Preparation System put you in charge of your exam by showing you test-taking strategies that work. Practice these strategies as you take the sample tests in this book, and then you will be ready to use them on test day.

First, you will take control of your time on the exam. The first step in achieving this control is to find out the format of the exam you're going to take. pharmacy technician exams will vary by state and may have different sections that are each timed separately. If this is true of the exam you will be taking, you will want to practice using your time wisely on the practice exams and try to avoid mistakes while working quickly. Other types of exams don't have separately timed sections. If this is the case, just practice pacing yourself on the practice exams so you don't spend too much time on difficult questions.

- **Listen carefully to directions.** By the time you get to the exam, you should know how the test works, but listen just in case something has changed.
- **Pace yourself.** Glance at your watch every few minutes, and compare the time to how far you've gotten in the section. Leave time for review, so that when one-quarter of the time has elapsed, you should be more than a quarter of the way through the section, and so on. If you're falling behind, pick up the pace a bit.
- **Keep moving.** Don't dither around on one question. If you don't know the answer, skip the question and move on. Circle the number of the question in your test booklet in case you have time to come back to it later.
- **Keep track of your place on the answer sheet.** If you skip a question, make sure you skip on the answer sheet, too. Check yourself every five to ten questions to make sure the question number and the answer sheet number are still the same.
- **Don't rush.** Though you should keep moving, rushing won't help. Try to keep calm and work methodically and quickly.

Step 5: Learn to Use the Process of Elimination

Time to complete: 20 minutes
Activity: Complete worksheet on Using the Process of Elimination
After time management, your next most important tool for taking control of your exam is using the process of elimination wisely. It's standard test-taking wisdom that you should always read all the answer choices before choosing your answer. This helps you find the right answer by eliminating wrong answer choices. And, sure enough, that standard wisdom applies to your exam, too.

Let's say you're facing a vocabulary question that goes like this:

13. "Biology uses a binomial system of classification." In this sentence, the word *binomial* most nearly means
   a. understanding the law.
   b. having two names.
   c. scientifically sound.
   d. having a double meaning.

If you happen to know what *binomial* means, you don't need to use the process of elimination, but let's assume that you don't. So, you look at the answer choices. *Understanding the law* sure doesn't sound very likely for something having to do with biology. So, you eliminate choice **a**—and now you only have three answer choices to deal with. Mark an X next to choice **a** so you never have to read it again.

Move on to the other answer choices. If you know that the prefix *bi-* means *two*, as in *bicycle*, you will flag answer **b** as a possible answer. Make a check mark beside it, meaning "good answer, I might use this one."

Choice **c**, *scientifically sound*, is a possibility. At least it's about science, not law. It could work here; though, when you think about it, having a *scientifically sound* classification system in a scientific field is kind of redundant. You remember the *bi-* in *binomial*, and probably continue to like answer **b** better. But you're not sure, so you put a question mark next to **c**, meaning "well, maybe."

Now, look at choice **d**, *having a double meaning*. You're still keeping in mind that *bi-* means *two*, so this one looks possible at first. But then you look again at the sentence the word belongs in, and you think, "Why would biology want a system of classification that has two meanings? That wouldn't work very well!" If you're really taken with the idea that *bi-* means *two*, you might put a question mark here. But if you're feeling a little more confident, you will put an X. You've already got a better answer picked out.

Now, your question looks like this:

13. "Biology uses a binomial system of classification." In this sentence, the word *binomial* most nearly means
  ✗ **a.** understanding the law.
  ✓ **b.** having two names.
  ? **c.** scientifically sound.
  ? **d.** having a double meaning.

You've got just one check mark, for a good answer. If you're pressed for time, you should simply mark answer **b** on your answer sheet. If you've got the time to be extra careful, you could compare your check mark answer to your question mark answers to make sure that it's better. (It is: The *binomial* system in biology is the one that gives a two-part genus and species a name like *homo sapiens*.)

It's good to have a system for marking good, bad, and maybe answers. We recommend using this one:

  ✗ = bad
  ✓ = good
  ? = maybe

If you don't like these marks, devise your own system. Just make sure you do it long before test day—while you're working through the practice in this book—so you won't have to worry about it during the test.

Even when you think you're absolutely clueless about a question, you can often use the process of elimination to get rid of one answer choice. If you do, you're better prepared to make an educated guess, as you will see in Step 6. More often, the process of elimination allows you to get down to only two possibly right answers. Then you're in a strong position to guess. And sometimes, even though you don't know the right answer, you find it simply by getting rid of the wrong ones, as you did in the example above.

Try using your powers of elimination on the questions in the worksheet Using the Process of Elimination beginning on page 16. The answer explanations there show one possible way you might use the process to arrive at the right answer.

The process of elimination is your tool for the next step, which is knowing when to guess.

Using the Process of Elimination

Use the process of elimination to answer the following questions.

1. Ilsa is as old as Meghan will be in five years. The difference between Ed's age and Meghan's age is twice the difference between Ilsa's age and Meghan's age. Ed is 29. How old is Ilsa?
   - a. 4
   - b. 10
   - c. 19
   - d. 24

2. "All drivers of commercial vehicles must carry a valid commercial driver's license whenever operating a commercial vehicle." According to this sentence, which of the following people need NOT carry a commercial driver's license?
   - a. a truck driver idling his engine while waiting to be directed to a loading dock
   - b. a bus operator backing her bus out of the way of another bus in the bus lot
   - c. a taxi driver driving his personal car to the grocery store
   - d. a limousine driver taking the limousine to her home after dropping off her last passenger of the evening

3. Smoking tobacco has been linked to
   - a. increased risk of stroke and heart attack.
   - b. all forms of respiratory disease.
   - c. increasing mortality rates over the past ten years.
   - d. juvenile delinquency.

4. Which of the following words is spelled correctly?
   - a. incorrigible
   - b. outragous
   - c. domestickated
   - d. understandible

Answers

Here are the answers, as well as some suggestions as to how you might have used the process of elimination to find them.

1. **d.** You should have eliminated answer **a** off the bat. Ilsa can't be four years old if Meghan is going to be Ilsa's age in five years. The best way to eliminate other answer choices is to try plugging them in to the information given in the problem. For instance, for answer **b**, if Ilsa is 10, then Meghan must be 5. The difference in their ages is 5. The difference between Ed's age, 29, and Meghan's age, 5, is 24. Is 24 two times 5? No. Then answer **b** is wrong. You could eliminate answer **c** in the same way and be left with answer **d**.

2. **c.** Note the word *not* in the question, and go through the answers one by one. Is the truck driver in choice **a** "operating a commercial vehicle"? Yes, idling counts as *operating*, so he needs to have a commercial driver's license. Likewise, the bus operator in answer **b** is operating a commercial vehicle; the question doesn't say the operator has to be on the

street. The limo driver in **d** is operating a commercial vehicle, even if it doesn't have a passenger in it. However, the cabbie in answer **c** is not operating a commercial vehicle, but his own private car.

3. a. You could eliminate answer **b** simply because of the presence of the word *all*. Such absolutes hardly ever appear in correct answer choices. Choice **c** looks attractive until you think a little about what you know—aren't fewer people smoking these days, rather than more? So how could smoking be responsible for a higher mortality rate? (If you didn't know that mortality rate means the rate at which people die, you might keep this choice as a possibility, but you'd still be able to eliminate two answers and have only two to choose from.) And choice **d** is plain silly, so you could eliminate that one, too. You're left with the correct answer, choice **a**.

4. a. How you used the process of elimination here depends on which words you recognized as being spelled incorrectly. If you knew that the correct spellings were *outrageous, domesticated,* and *understandable,* then you were home free. Surely you knew that at least one of those words was wrong!

Step 6: Know When to Guess

Time to complete: 20 minutes
Activity: Complete worksheet on Your Guessing Ability

Armed with the process of elimination, you're ready to take control of one of the big questions in test taking: Should I guess?

The first and main answer is "Yes." Unless the exam has a so-called guessing penalty, you have nothing to lose and everything to gain from guessing. More complicated answers depend both on the exam and on you—your personality and your "guessing intuition."

Most pharmacy technology exams don't use a guessing penalty. The number of questions you answer correctly yields your score, and there's no penalty for wrong answers. So most of the time, you don't have to worry—simply go ahead and guess. But if you find that your exam does have a guessing penalty, you should read the section below to find out what that means to you.

How the Guessing Penalty Works

A guessing penalty really only works against random guessing—filling in the little circles to make a nice pattern on your answer sheet. If you can eliminate one or more answer choices, as outlined above, you're better off taking a guess than leaving the answer blank, even on the sections that have a penalty.

Here's how a guessing penalty works: Depending on the number of answer choices in a given exam, some proportion of the number of questions you get wrong is subtracted from the total number of questions you got right. For instance, if there are four answer choices, typically the guessing penalty is one-third of your wrong answers.

Suppose you took a test of 100 questions. You answered 88 of them right and 12 wrong. If there's no guessing penalty, your score is simply 88. But if there's a one-third point guessing penalty, the scorers take your 12 wrong answers and divide by 3 to come up with 4. Then they subtract that 4 from your correct-answer score of 88 to leave you with a score of 84. Thus, you would have been better off if you had simply not answered those 12 questions that you weren't sure of—your total score would still be 88 because there wouldn't be anything to subtract.

What You Should Do about the Guessing Penalty

You now know how a guessing penalty works. The first thing this means for you is that marking your answer sheet at random doesn't pay. If you're running out of time on an exam that has a guessing penalty, you should not use your remaining seconds to mark a pretty pattern on your answer sheet. Take those few seconds to try to answer one more question right.

But as soon as you get out of the realm of random guessing, the guessing penalty no longer works against you. If you can use the process of elimination to get rid of even one wrong answer choice, the odds stop being against you and start working in your favor.

Sticking with our example of an exam that has four answer choices, eliminating just one wrong answer makes your odds of choosing the correct answer one in three. That's the same as the one-third point guessing penalty we previously mentioned—even odds. If you eliminate two answer choices, your odds are one in two—better than our guessing penalty. In either case, you should go ahead and choose one of the remaining answer choices.

When There Is No Guessing Penalty

As noted above, most pharmacy technology exams don't have a guessing penalty. That means that, all other things being equal, you should always go ahead and guess, even if you have no idea what the question means. Nothing can happen to you if you're wrong. But all other things aren't necessarily equal. The other factor in deciding whether or not to guess, besides the guessing penalty, is you. There are two things you need to know about yourself before you go into the exam:

1. Are you a risk-taker?
2. Are you a good guesser?

Your risk-taking temperament matters most on exams with a guessing penalty. Without a guessing penalty, even if you're a play-it-safe person, guessing is perfectly safe. Overcome your anxieties, and go ahead and mark an answer.

But what if you're not much of a risk-taker, and you think of yourself as the world's worst guesser? Complete the following worksheet Your Guessing Ability to get an idea of how good your intuition is.

Your Guessing Ability

The following are ten really hard questions. You're not supposed to know the answers. Rather, this is an assessment of your ability to guess when you don't have a clue. Read each question carefully, as if you were expected to answer them. If you have any knowledge at all of the subject of the question, use that knowledge to help you eliminate wrong answer choices.

1. September 7 is Independence Day in
   a. India.
   b. Costa Rica.
   c. Brazil.
   d. Australia.

2. Which of the following is the formula for determining the momentum of an object?
   a. $p = mv$
   b. $F = ma$
   c. $P = IV$
   d. $E = mc^2$

3. Because of the expansion of the universe, the stars and other celestial bodies are all moving away from each other. This phenomenon is known as
   a. Newton's first law.
   b. the Big Bang.
   c. gravitational collapse.
   d. Hubble flow.

4. American author Gertrude Stein was born in
   a. 1713.
   b. 1830.
   c. 1874.
   d. 1901.

5. Which of the following is NOT one of the Five Classics attributed to Confucius?
   a. the *I Ching*
   b. the *Book of Holiness*
   c. the *Spring and Autumn Annals*
   d. the *Book of History*

6. The religious and philosophical doctrine that holds that the universe is constantly in a struggle between good and evil is known as
   a. Pelagianism.
   b. Manichaeanism.
   c. neo-Hegelianism.
   d. Epicureanism.

7. The third chief justice of the U.S. Supreme Court was
   a. John Blair.
   b. William Cushing.
   c. James Wilson.
   d. John Jay.

8. Which of the following is the poisonous portion of a daffodil?
   a. the bulb
   b. the leaves
   c. the stem
   d. the flowers

9. The winner of the Masters Golf Tournament in 1953 was
   a. Sam Snead.
   b. Cary Middlecoff.
   c. Arnold Palmer.
   d. Ben Hogan.

10. The state with the highest per capita personal income in 1980 was
    a. Alaska.
    b. Connecticut.
    c. New York.
    d. Texas.

Answers

Check your answers against the correct answers below.

1. c.
2. a.
3. d.
4. c.
5. b.
6. b.
7. b.
8. a.
9. d.
10. a.

How Did You Do?

You may have simply gotten lucky and actually known the answer to one or two questions. In addition, your guessing was more successful if you were able to use the process of elimination on any of the questions. Maybe you didn't know who the third chief justice was (question 7), but you knew that John Jay was the first. In that case, you would have eliminated answer **d** and, therefore, improved your odds of guessing right from one in four to one in three.

According to probability, you should get two and a half answers correct, so getting either two or three right would be average. If you got four or more right, you may be a really terrific guesser. If you got one or none right, you may be a really bad guesser.

Keep in mind, though, that this is only a small sample. You should continue to keep track of your guessing ability as you work through the sample questions in this book. Circle the number of questions you guessed on as you answer; or, if you don't have time while you take the practice tests, go back afterward and try to remember which questions you guessed at. Remember, on a test with four answer choices, your chances of getting a right answer is one in four. So keep a separate guessing score for each exam. How many questions did you guess on? How many did you get right? If the number you got right is at least one-fourth of the number of questions you guessed on, you are at least an average guesser, maybe better—and you should always go ahead and guess on the real exam. If the number you got right is significantly lower than one-fourth of the number you guessed on, you need to improve your guessing skills.

Step 7: Reach Your Peak Performance Zone

Time to complete: 10 minutes to read; weeks to complete!
Activity: Complete the Physical Preparation Checklist

To get ready for a challenge like a big exam, you have to take control of your physical, as well as your mental, state. Exercise, proper diet, and rest will ensure that your body works with, rather than against, your mind on test day, as well as during your preparation.

Exercise

If you don't already have a regular exercise program going, the time during which you're preparing for an exam is actually an excellent time to start one. And if you're already keeping fit—or trying to get that way—don't let the pressure of preparing for an exam fool you into quitting now. Exercise helps reduce stress by pumping wonderful good-feeling hormones called endorphins into your system. It also increases the oxygen supply throughout your body, including to your brain, so you will be at peak performance on test day.

A half hour of vigorous activity—enough to raise a sweat—every day should be your aim. If you're really pressed for time, every other day is OK. Choose an activity you like and get out there and do it. Jogging with a friend always makes the time go faster, or take a radio or MP3 player.

But don't overdo it. You don't want to exhaust yourself. Moderation is the key.

Diet

First of all, cut out the junk. Go easy on caffeine and nicotine, and eliminate alcohol and any other drugs from your system at least two weeks before the exam. Promise yourself a party the night after the exam, if need be.

What your body needs for peak performance is simply a balanced diet. Eat plenty of fruits and vegetables, along with protein and carbohydrates. Foods that are high in lecithin (an amino acid), such as fish and beans, are especially good "brain foods."

The night before the exam, you might "carbo-load" the way athletes do before a contest. Eat a big plate of spaghetti, rice and beans, or whatever your favorite carbohydrate is.

Rest

You probably know how much sleep you need every night to be at your best, even if you don't always get it. Make sure you do get that much sleep, though, for at least a week before the exam. Moderation is important here, too. Too much sleep will just make you groggy.

If you're not a morning person and your exam will be given in the morning, you should reset your internal clock so that your body doesn't think you're taking an exam at 3 A.M. You have to start this process well before the exam. Get up half an hour earlier each morning, and then go to bed half an hour earlier that night. Don't try it the other way around; you will just toss and turn if you go to bed early without having gotten up early. The next morning, get up another half an hour earlier, and so on. The length of this process depends on how late you're used to getting up. Use the Physical Preparation Checklist on the next page to make sure you're in tip-top form.

Physical Preparation Checklist

For the week before the exam, write down (1) what physical exercise you engaged in and for how long and (2) what you ate for each meal. Remember, you're trying for at least half an hour of exercise every other day (preferably every day) and a balanced diet that's light on junk food.

Exam minus 7 days

Exercise: _____ for _____ minutes

Breakfast: _____

Lunch: _____

Dinner: _____

Snacks: _____

Exam minus 6 days

Exercise: _____ for _____ minutes

Breakfast: _____

Lunch: _____

Dinner: _____

Snacks: _____

Exam minus 5 days

Exercise: _____ for _____ minutes

Breakfast: _____

Lunch: _____

Dinner: _____

Snacks: _____

Exam minus 4 days

Exercise: _____ for _____ minutes

Breakfast: _____

Lunch: _____

Dinner: _____

Snacks: _____

Exam minus 3 days

Exercise: _____ for _____ minutes

Breakfast: _____

Lunch: _____

Dinner: _____

Snacks: _____

Exam minus 2 days

Exercise: _____ for _____ minutes

Breakfast: _____

Lunch: _____

Dinner: _____

Snacks: _____

Exam minus 1 day

Exercise: _____ for _____ minutes

Breakfast: _____

Lunch: _____

Dinner: _____

Snacks: _____

Step 8: Get Your Act Together

Time to complete: 10 minutes to read; time to complete will vary
Activity: Complete Final Preparations worksheet (page 24)
You're in control of your mind and body; you're in charge of test anxiety, your preparation, and your test-taking strategies. Now, it's time to take charge of external factors, like the testing site and the materials you need to take the exam.

Find Out Where the Test Is and Make a Trial Run

The testing agency or your pharmacy technology instructor will notify you when and where your exam is being held. Do you know how to get to the testing site? Do you know how long it will take to get there? If not, make a trial run, preferably on the same day of the week at the same time of day. Make note, on the worksheet on page 24, of the amount of time it will take you to get to the exam site. Plan on arriving 10–15 minutes early so you can get the lay of the land, use the bathroom, and calm down. Then figure out how early you will have to get up that morning, and make sure you get up that early every day for a week before the exam.

Gather Your Materials

The night before the exam, lay out the clothes you will wear and the materials you have to bring with you to the exam. Plan on dressing in layers; you won't have any control over the temperature of the examination room. Have a sweater or jacket you can take off if it's warm. Use the checklist on the following Final Preparations worksheet to help you pull together what you will need.

Don't Skip Breakfast

Even if you don't usually eat breakfast, do so on exam morning. A cup of coffee doesn't count. Don't do doughnuts or other sweet foods, either. A sugar high will leave you with a sugar low in the middle of the exam. A mix of protein and carbohydrates is best: cereal with milk and just a little sugar or eggs with toast will do your body a world of good.

Final Preparations

Getting to the Exam Site

Location of exam site: _____

Date: _____

Departure time: _____

Do I know how to get to the exam site? Yes _____ No _____   If no, make a trial run.

Time it will take to get to exam site: _____

Things to Lay Out the Night Before

Clothes I will wear _____

Sweater/jacket _____

Watch _____

Photo ID _____

No. 2 pencils _____

Other Things to Bring/Remember

_____   _____

_____   _____

_____   _____

_____   _____

Step 9: Do It!

Time to complete: 10 minutes, plus test-taking time

Activity: Ace the pharmacy technician exam!

Fast forward to exam day. You're ready. You made a study plan and followed through. You practiced your test-taking strategies while working through this book. You're in control of your physical, mental, and emotional state. You know when and where to show up and what to bring with you. In other words, you're better prepared than most of the other people taking the pharmacy technician national exam with you. You're psyched!

Just one more thing. When you're done with the exam, you will have earned a reward. Plan a celebration. Call up your friends and plan a party, or have a nice dinner for two—whatever your heart desires. Give yourself something to look forward to.

And then do it. Go into the exam, full of confidence, armed with test-taking strategies you've practiced until they're second nature. You're in control of yourself, your environment, and your performance on the exam. You're ready to succeed. So do it. Go in there and ace the exam. And look forward to your future career as a pharmacy technician!

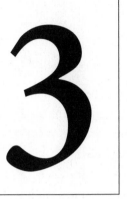

3 ▶ Diagnostic Test

CHAPTER OVERVIEW
This practice diagnostic test is based on information you will need to know when taking either of the pharmacy technician national exams or an individual state or employer exam. Of course, none of these questions and answers is reproduced from an actual pharmacy technician exam, due to copyright restrictions, but this test does offer the information needed and also in the same format as you will find on either national exams offered.

This practice diagnostic test is modeled on the PTCB exam and contains 90 multiple-choice questions to be completed in 110 minutes. It is important to make sure you time yourself to ensure that you are practicing under conditions similar to the actual test.

Before taking this test, study Chapter 2: The LearningExpress Test Preparation System to help you develop the skills needed to succeed on the pharmacy technician exam and any future tests you may encounter in any field.

Please use the answer sheet on the following page. Once you have completed the test in the allotted time, go to the Answers and Explanations on page 37, and count the number of questions you answered correctly. Make note of the questions you answered incorrectly, as you will want to concentrate your review on those subjects.

Practice Questions

1. What type of tip will you find on a syringe meant to hold a needle in place?
   a. luer lock
   b. glass
   c. slip-tip
   d. reusable

2. Of the following drug classifications, which one would the drug fluoxetine be found in?
   a. H2 blockers
   b. beta-blockers
   c. SSRI
   d. ACE inhibitors

3. Which category of drug would be indicated for the treatment of pain?
   a. antitussive
   b. analgesic
   c. antipyretic
   d. antihyperlipidemic

4. Tenormin® or atenolol would be in what classification of drug?
   a. proton pump inhibitors
   b. A2 receptor antagonists
   c. ACE inhibitors
   d. beta-blockers

5. There are rules that regulate the refilling of controlled drugs. Of the following drugs, which one cannot be refilled under any circumstance?
   a. hydrocodone/acetaminophen
   b. diazepam
   c. oxycodone
   d. propoxyphene/acetaminophen

6. Calculate the flow rate in drops per minute if a physician orders D5W/NS 1,000 ml over 12 hours, with an administration set that delivers 16 gtt/ml.
   a. 17 gtt/min
   b. 22 gtt/min
   c. 30 gtt/min
   d. 44 gtt/min

7. The labeling of legend drug containers will generally have two names on them, the generic and the trade or brand name. What exactly is the trade or brand name?
   a. the common name of the drug
   b. the name the drug manufacturer gives the drug
   c. the chemical name of the drug
   d. the abbreviated generic name of the drug

8. A physician special-orders 120 g of 1.5% hydrocortisone cream. The pharmacy stocks 2.5% and 1% hydrocortisone creams. How much of each stock item will a technician need to prepare this compound correctly?
   a. 80 g of 1% and 40 g of 2.5%
   b. 60 g of each strength
   c. 80 g of 2.5% and 40 g of 2.5%
   d. 90 g of 1% and 30 g of 2.5%

9. Medications that are prepackaged into unit doses must have what information included on the label?
   a. patient's name, dispense date, medication name, and directions for use
   b. medication name and strength, lot number, and directions for use
   c. directions for use, medication name and strength, expiration date
   d. medication name and strength, lot number, and expiration date

10. In which class of controlled medications is Percocet® found, as indicated by the Controlled Substances Act (CSA)?
  a. schedule I
  b. schedule II
  c. schedule III
  d. schedule IV

11. The following prescription is brought to the pharmacy: "Amoxil® suspension 400 mg po tid × 10 days." The pharmacy stocks 500/5 ml amoxicillin suspension. What is the volume of medication needed to fill the entire prescription?
  a. 60 ml
  b. 120 ml
  c. 240 ml
  d. 30 ml

12. Of the following solutions, which one is the least concentrated?
  a. 1:100
  b. 1:500
  c. 1:1,000
  d. 1:1,500

13. A technician takes a phone call from a patient complaining that she didn't feel well a few hours after taking a new medication. She wants to know what the side effects are for her new medication. What should the technician do?
  a. Ask the patient to hold while he or she looks up the side effects in a reference book.
  b. Tell the patient to lie down and wait for the side effects to wear off.
  c. Put the patient on hold and notify the pharmacist of the situation.
  d. Tell the patient what the side effects are, since they are commonly known.

14. The retail price of a prescription is based on AWP, plus a markup and a dispensing fee. Use the table below to determine the retail price of a prescription of 20 tablets, if a bottle of 100 has an AWP of $49.70 and a markup of 6%.

AWP	Dispensing Fee
$0–$5.00	$4.40
$5.01–$10.00	$5.40
$10.01–$20.00	$6.40
$20.00 and up	$7.40

  a. $11.94
  b. $15.34
  c. $9.94
  d. $15.94

15. How many 500 mg metronidazole tablets are needed to compound the following prescription: "metronidazole 6% 150 ml"?
  a. 18
  b. 16
  c. 8
  d. 4

16. In the NDC number, 00093-4150-10, what do the numbers "10" identify?
  a. manufacturer
  b. package size
  c. product
  d. strength

17. Which of the following medications is classified as an A2 receptor antagonist?
  a. glipizide
  b. enalapril
  c. losartan
  d. atenolol

18. How many tablets will it take to fill the following prescription as it is written?

amoxicillin 250 mg
i po tid × 14 days

a. 46
b. 42
c. 18
d. 53

19. The portion paid by a patient, who has insurance, for a retail prescription is known as the
a. co-payment.
b. deductible.
c. premium.
d. tip.

20. What is the total volume of fluid needed if D5W is to run at 25 ml/hr for 24 hours?
a. 425
b. 500
c. 250
d. 600

21. The doctor orders codeine gr $\frac{1}{4}$. How many milligrams is this equal to?
a. 15
b. 30
c. 60
d. 90

22. How much dextrose would be found in a D5W 1,000 ml IV bag?
a. There are 5 g of dextrose in this bag.
b. There are 50 g of dextrose in this bag.
c. There are 250 g of dextrose in this bag.
d. There are 500 g of dextrose in this bag.

23. What is the proper temperature for storing an item in the refrigerator?
a. less than 36 degrees Fahrenheit
b. 2 to 8 degrees Celsius
c. 15 to 30 degrees Celsius
d. 59 to 86 degrees Fahrenheit

24. Which of the following medications listed is an H1 blocker?
a. loratidine
b. cimetidine
c. nifedipine
d. ranitidine

25. Which of the following drug classes indicates there is a strong likelihood that the drug will cause serious adverse effects or death?
a. class I
b. class II
c. class III
d. class IV

26. Which of the following concepts refers to the protection of identity and health information of patients?
a. morality
b. mortality
c. motility
d. confidentiality

27. A patient needs KCL 5 mEq IV. The pharmacy stocks 20 mEq/ml in a 5 ml multi-dose vial. What will be the volume needed to provide the correct dose?
a. 4 ml
b. 0.25 ml
c. 5 ml
d. 0.5 ml

28. According to federal law, what is the maximum number of refills permitted for a schedule IV controlled substance?
   a. 6 refills in six months
   b. 11 refills in one year
   c. 5 refills in six months
   d. no refills allowed

29. What is the trade name for metformin?
   a. Glucophage®
   b. Micronase®
   c. Glucotrol®
   d. Diabinese®

30. 240 ml of a zithromax 5% suspension contains how many milligrams of active ingredient?
   a. 12 mg
   b. 120 mg
   c. 1,200 mg
   d. 12,000 mg

31. The pharmacy has 10% strength and 2% strength of a certain ointment. A patient brings in a prescription for 6 oz of this ointment, but in 7.5% strength. Which of the following would be needed to compound the ointment?
   a. 47.25 g of 10% and 131.75 g of 2%
   b. 50 g of 2% and 130 g of 10%
   c. 123.75 g of 10% and 56.25 g of 2%
   d. 130 g of 10% and 50 g of 2%

32. Which of the following medications is an H2 antagonist?
   a. loratidine
   b. hyoscyamine
   c. ranitidine
   d. clonidine

33. Gentamicin injection is given to a patient at 5 mg/kg/day in three divided doses. If a patient weighs 144 lb, what would be the approximate strength of a single dose?
   a. 109 mg
   b. 110 mg
   c. 327 mg
   d. none of the above

34. If a patient calls for refills of their Tenormin® and Glucotrol®, which of the following combinations of medications would be needed to fill the order?
   a. enalapril and metformin
   b. atenolol and glyburide
   c. atenolol and glipizide
   d. enalapril and glipizide

35. How many 125 mg doses of Vancocin® can be withdrawn from a 1 g vial?
   a. eight doses
   b. six doses
   c. nine doses
   d. four doses

36. Which of the following needles has the largest bore or diameter?
   a. 29 gauge
   b. 16 gauge
   c. 27 gauge
   d. 23 gauge

37. The laminar flow hood should remain on at all times. If it is shut off, how long must it be left on before pharmacy staff can compound products in it?
   a. 45 minutes
   b. one hour
   c. 15 minutes
   d. 30 minutes

38. Identify which of the following sig codes correctly indicates the following directions: Take one tablet every six hours as needed.
a. 1 tab qid prn
b. 1 cap q6h prn
c. 1 tab q6h pp
d. 1 tab q6h prn

39. How many milliliters of a 1:250 stock solution will be needed approximately to make 240 ml of a 1:5,000 solution?
a. 6
b. 12
c. 18
d. 24

40. A patient with an allergy to amoxicillin will most likely have a sensitivity to what else?
a. gentamycin
b. erythromycin
c. cephalexin
d. tetracycline

41. How many ounces are equal to 12 kg?
a. 4
b. 40
c. 400
d. 1,200

42. When a liquid is added to a powder formulation such as an oral antibiotic suspension, what do we call this?
a. trituration
b. levigation
c. reconstitution
d. mixation

43. Na is the chemical symbol for which of the following elements?
a. nitrogen
b. sodium
c. nickel
d. aluminum

44. The practice of pharmacy is regulated by both federal and state law. Which one of the following federal laws mandates the use of safety caps?
a. FD&C act
b. PPPA
c. HIPPA
d. OSHA

45. The approximate size container for the dispensing of 180 ml of liquid medication would be?
a. two ounces
b. four ounces
c. six ounces
d. eight ounces

46. A prescription reading "i-ii tabs qid prn pain" should have directions that state:
a. Take one or two tablets every six hours as needed.
b. Take one or two tablets four times a day as needed.
c. Take one or two tablets every six hours as needed for pain.
d. Take one or two tablets four times a day as needed for pain.

47. A physician writes an order for a patient to receive KCl 40 mEq/L NS. It is to be infused at a rate of 60 ml/hr. How much KCl will the patient receive in one hour?
a. 2.4 mEq
b. 2.5 mEq
c. 10 mEq
d. 5 mEq

48. To ensure that a laminar flow hood is working properly, how often should it be inspected?
a. every six months
b. every two years
c. every one month
d. every one year

49. The classification of drug H2 blockers work by
   a. neutralizing acid secretion.
   b. inhibiting acid secretion.
   c. inhibiting stomach smooth muscles.
   d. decreasing peristalsis of the GI tract.

50. A pharmacy receives an order for 10% ointment. The pharmacy only stocks 15% and 5% strengths of this ointment. In what ratio should the two stock ointments be mixed in order to properly compound the prescription?
   a. 2:1
   b. 1:3
   c. 1:2
   d. 1:1

51. When withdrawing medication from an ampule, what size filter is needed to ensure any glass that may have fallen into the solution is filtered out?
   a. 0.5 micron
   b. 2 microns
   c. 5 microns
   d. 0.2 micron

52. The establishment of the Omnibus Budget Reconciliation Act (OBRA) in 1990 led to most states requiring which of the following?
   a. the use of pharmacy technicians
   b. the counseling of patients by pharmacists
   c. the enactment of the Controlled Substances Act
   d. inventory management of each pharmacy setting

53. One requirement of recertification is that the pharmacy technician must participate in how much continuing education?
   a. 10 contact hours every year
   b. 20 contact hours every year
   c. 10 contact hours every two years
   d. 20 contact hours every two years

54. What size hypodermic syringe should you use to give a 3.4 ml dose?
   a. 1 ml
   b. 3 ml
   c. 5 ml
   d. 10 ml

55. If a patient receives a medication at 5 mg/kg/day, what would a single dose be if the patient weighs 142 lb?
   a. approximately 150 mg
   b. approximately 323 mg
   c. approximately 161 mg
   d. approximately 80 mg

56. Of the following organ systems, which one is associated with the term *antitussive*?
   a. endocrine system
   b. gastrointestinal system
   c. respiratory system
   d. urinary system

57. You have dextrose 70% water 1,000 ml. How many kg of dextrose would you find in 400 ml of this solution?
   a. 280 kg
   b. 28 kg
   c. 2.8 kg
   d. 0.28 kg

58. Little Joey cannot swallow his 0.5 g tablet, so the pharmacy will compound the following suspension for him: 125 mg/5 ml 360 ml. How many 500 mg tablets will be needed to compound this?
   a. 8
   b. 18
   c. 26
   d. 32

59. How many grams of 2% hydrocortisone cream will deliver 1 g of active ingredient?
    a. 25 g
    b. 4 g
    c. 50 g
    d. 20 g

60. When storing an item at room temperature, how warm should the room be?
    a. 36 to 46 degrees Fahrenheit
    b. greater than 30 degrees Celsius
    c. 2 to 8 degrees Celsius
    d. 15 to 30 degrees Celsius

61. What schedule of controlled substances does zolpidem fall under?
    a. schedule III
    b. schedule II
    c. schedule IV
    d. schedule V

62. What is the list of medications called that a physician can prescribe within a given setting?
    a. MSDS
    b. a formulary
    c. an open system
    d. a closed panel of drugs

63. Which of the following sig codes indicates the following directions: "Take one teaspoon after meals as needed"?
    a. 1 tsp ac prn
    b. 1 tbsp ac prn
    c. 1 tsp pc prn
    d. 1 tbsp pc prn

64. Protocols established in your pharmacy setting can be found where?
    a. pharmacy reference book
    b. pharmacy policy and procedures manual
    c. *Facts and Comparisons*
    d. *Pharmacy Protocol Manual* (PPM)

65. What is the purpose of using an IVPB?
    a. for fluid replacement
    b. for fluid and electrolyte replacement
    c. for the delivery of medications needed
    d. to allow the LVP or SVP to run effectively

66. A laminar flow hood should be cleaned using side-to-side motions from
    a. the front of the hood to the back toward the HEPA filter.
    b. the back of the hood to the front away from the HEPA filter.
    c. up and down from the top of the hood to the bottom of the hood starting in back.
    d. up and down from the top of the hood to the bottom of the hood starting in front.

67. How many 1 L bags will be needed if D5W is to run 80 ml/hr for 24 hours?
    a. one bag
    b. two bags
    c. three bags
    d. four or more bags

68. You have Ceclor® 250 mg/5 ml 200 ml. How many milliliters needed to give a dose of 400 mg?
    a. two
    b. four
    c. six
    d. eight

69. If the dose in question number 68 is "400 mg po q8h × 10 days," what is the total volume needed to last the full ten days?
    a. 100 ml
    b. 140 ml
    c. 200 ml
    d. 240 ml

70. Which drug would be found in the classification of drugs called benzodiazepines?
a. zolpidem
b. metoprolol
c. alprazolam
d. azithromycin

71. If a pharmacy wanted to make a 30% profit on an item that was $5.75, what would the retail price need to be?
a. $1.72
b. $1.73
c. $7.48
d. $2.25

72. How many teaspoons are in a tablespoon?
a. two
b. three
c. four
d. five

73. How many tablets are needed for the following directions?

vi po bid × 2d, iv po bid × 2d, ii po qd × 2d then dc

a. 24
b. 34
c. 44
d. 54

74. At what distance within the laminar flow hood must all manipulations be performed?
a. 6 inches
b. 4 inches
c. 12 inches
d. 8 inches

75. Which form is used to order CII narcotics?
a. DEA Form 220
b. DEA Form 121
c. DEA Form 222
d. DEA Form 200

76. Which medication is classified as a calcium channel blocker?
a. nitroglycerin
b. enalapril
c. atenolol
d. amlodipine

77. Which DEA number would not be valid for Dr. George Carswell?
a. BC3421234
b. AC6782329
c. AC3081421
d. AC1355672

78. Which of the following medications is used to regulate the level of fluid in the body?
a. anti-inflammatory
b. antipyretic
c. diuretic
d. benzodiazepine

79. *The Orange Book* is most commonly used to find what?
a. direct prices
b. manufacturers' standards
c. therapeutic equivalence
d. generic equivalence

80. The HEPA filter, which is part of the laminar flow hood, is used to remove particle sizes less than
a. 5 microns.
b. 0.2 microns.
c. 2 microns.
d. 0.5 microns.

81. You receive an order for cefazolin eye drops 1:1,000 solution 10 ml. How many milligrams of cefazolin are needed to prepare these eye drops?
a. two
b. four
c. eight
d. ten

82. A patient would like information concerning a good decongestant that is available over-the-counter (OTC). What should you do?
    a. Show them the antihistamines available in the cold section and let them make a choice.
    b. Inform them of which one you use and recommend it.
    c. Inform the patient that they should talk with the pharmacist.
    d. Find out if the patient has any allergies—and if not, direct them to the cold medication section of the pharmacy.

83. Vicodin® is the same as
    a. acetaminophen with codeine.
    b. hydrocodone with codeine.
    c. oxycodone with acetaminophen.
    d. hydrocodone with acetaminophen.

84. Approximately how many gr 5 tablets are needed for a dose of 1.2 g?
    a. four
    b. five
    c. six
    d. seven

85. An antibiotic injection given in a small volume of solution that is connected to a main line IV is commonly known as an
    a. IV piggyback.
    b. IV push.
    c. IV injection.
    d. IV transfusion.

86. A pharmacy has 200 ml of a 1:50 solution in stock. If the technician dilutes the solution to 500 ml, what will be the final strength of the solution?
    a. 8%
    b. 0.8%
    c. 4%
    d. 0.04%

87. Of the following reference books, which one would be the most updated?
    a. *Facts and Comparisons*
    b. *Physician's Desk Reference* (PDR)
    c. *Remington's Pharmaceutical Sciences*
    d. *United States Pharmacopoeia Drug Information* (USPDI)

88. How much hydrocortisone powder would be present in two ounces of 1% hydrocortisone cream?
    a. 0.2 g
    b. 0.6 g
    c. 0.8 g
    d. 1.2 g

89. A patient is on an insulin regimen of 40 units SC q am and 35 units SC q pm. How many vials will be needed to last 30 days?
    a. one vial
    b. two vials
    c. three vials
    d. four or more vials

90. Which of these products is not time-release?
    a. Inderal LA®
    b. Robitussin DM®
    c. Contact TR®
    d. Theodur SA®

Answers and Explanations

1. a. A luer lock tip syringe allows a needle to be screwed in place to ensure the needle stays in place. A syringe without a luer lock tip will always leave the possibility of the needle slipping off.

2. c. Fluoxetine is in the classification of drug we call serotonin-specific reuptake inhibitors (SSRI), which are used in the treatment of depression.

3. b. Analgesics are medications that relieve pain, antitussives would be used for cough, antipyretics would be used for fever, and hyperlipidemics would be used for high cholesterol.

4. d. Atenolol is a beta-blocker. In most cases, you know this because the ending of a generic drug in this classification usually ends in -*olol*.

5. c. Oxycodone is a schedule II controlled substance. Under current law, a CII prescription cannot be written with refills—or if so, refills cannot be given.

6. b. Use ratio and proportion. Setup: 1,000 ml/12 hr = x ml/1 min, which will need to be changed so units match on the top and bottom of this proportion: 1,000 ml/720 min = x ml/1 min, x = 1.39 ml/min. Setup for step 2: (1.39 ml/min) (16 gtts/ml) = 22 gtts/min.

7. b. The National Drug Code (NDC) number gives us information for each set of numbers in it. The first set tells us who the manufacturer is, the second set tells us the drug product, and the third set is the package size.

8. a. Using the allegation chart, you get 0.5/1.5 × 120 = 40 g of the 2.5% and 1/1.5 × 120 = 80 g of the 1%.

9. d. When prepackaging, it must indicate medication name and strength, lot number to track specific batches of the medication, and expiration date to indicate the window of use.

10. b. Percocet®, or oxycodone with acetaminophen, is a schedule II drug. Schedule II drugs are considered to have the highest abuse potential of all drugs in the pharmacy.

11. b. Use ratio and proportion. Individual Dose setup: 400 mg/x ml = 500 mg/5 ml, x = 4 ml; then just insert your individual dose into the directions and multiply for total volume needed: (4 ml)(3)(10) = 120 ml.

12. d. 1:1,500, because there is only 1 g of active drug per 1,500 ml of (solvent) solution. If we look at the other ratios, we see less solvent (solution) per 1 g active drug which makes them more concentrated.

13. c. Any role that requires a judgmental decision should be done by the pharmacist. This would include counseling.

14. d. Prescription pricing in this case involves the AWP + markup + dispensing fee. $49.70/100 = x/20 = $9.94; plus markup of $0.60 + $5.40 (dispensing fee) = $15.94.

15. a. Use ratio and proportion first to find the total amount of the drug needed. Setup: 6 g/100 ml = x g/150 ml, x = 9 g. Then find how many tablets you need to make. Setup: 1 tab/500 mg = x tabs/9,000 mg, x = 18 tablets.

16. b. The last two digits in the NDC indicate the size of the package. The first set of digits is the manufacturer, and the third set would be the package size.

17. c. Losartan is an A2 receptor antagonist. Glipizide is a sulfonylurea. Enalapril is an ACE inhibitor. Atenolol is a beta-blocker.

18. b. (One tab) (3 times per day) (14 days) = 42 tabs.

19. a. In the case of third-party prescriptions, the patient has insurance and only needs to pay a minimal fee or co-payment. The pharmacy in turn will bill the insurance company, less the co-payment.

20. d. Use ratio and proportion. Setup: 25 ml/1 hr = x ml/24 hr = x = 600 ml.

21. a. Use ratio and proportion. Setup: gr 1/60 mg = gr $\frac{1}{4}$/x mg; x = 15 mg.

22. b. Use ratio and proportion. Setup: 5 g/100 ml = x g/1,000 ml; x = 50 g.

23. b. Two to 8 degrees Celsius is equal to 36 to 46 degrees Fahrenheit, which is the required temperature for refrigerated storage.

24. a. Loratidine, the generic version of Zyrtec®, is an H1 or histamine 1 blocker, or antagonist; cimetidine and ranitidine are both H2 blockers; nifedipine is a calcium channel blocker.

25. a. There are three classes of drug recalls. Class I is the most serious, with potential for adverse effects or death. Class II drugs have the potential for adverse effects, but not as serious as class I. No harmful adverse effects are associated with a class III recall.

26. d. Confidentiality is the concept of protecting information. It is an important part of HIPAA, which regulates the need for patient confidentiality.

27. b. Use ratio and proportion. Setup: 20 mEq/1 ml = 5 mEq/x ml; x = 0.25 ml.

28. c. A CIV controlled prescription is only valid for a period of six months. During that time, a patient can only refill it five times. This also applies to all controlled drugs that are CIII through CV. CII drugs cannot have any refills.

29. a. The trade name for metformin is Glucophage®, Micronase® would be glyburide, Glucotrol® would be glipizide, and Diabinese® would be chlorpropamide.

30. d. Use ratio and proportion. Setup: 5,000 mg/100 ml = x mg/240 ml; x = 12,000 mg.

31. c. 5.5/8 × 180 = 123.75 g of 10%; 2.5/8 × 180 = 56.25 g of 2%.

32. c. Ranitidine is in the classification of drug we call an H2 blocker or antagonist.

33. a. Use ratio and proportion. Setup: 5 mg/2.2 lb = x mg/144 lb; x = 327.5 mg per day, but this is the total daily dose, so you need to divide by 3. 327.5 mg/3 = 109.1 mg.

34. c. The generic name for Tenormin® is atenolol, and the generic name for Glucotrol® is glipizide.

35. a. Use ratio and proportion. Setup: 1 dose/125 mg = 1,000 mg/x doses; x = 8 doses.

36. b. The smaller the gauge number, the larger the bore, or diameter.

37. d. The laminar flow hood must be turned off for a minimum of 30 minutes and then cleaned before use.

38. d. Indicates one tablet every six hours as needed.

39. b. Use ratio and proportion. Setup: 1 g/5,000 ml = x g/240 ml, x = 0.048 g. New setup: 1 g/250 ml = 0.048 g/x ml, x = 11.52 ml.

40. c. Cephalexin is related to penicillin, which may cause a patient to be more sensitive to this class of medication. If this is the case, this is known as cross-sensitivity. The protocol for those allergic to penicillin is to give them a macrolide antibiotic, such as erythromycin.

41. c. Use ratio and proportion. Setup: 1 oz/30 g = x oz/12,000 g, x = 400 g.

42. c. Reconstitution involves placing a solvent (liquid or solution) in a powdered formulation. Trituration means grinding a drug into a finer particle size using a mortar and pestle. And levigation is the same as trituration, but adding a small amount of liquid as well.

43. b. On the periodic table, Na is the symbol for sodium. This is often used when we refer to sodium chloride, or NaCl.

44. b. The Poison Prevention Packaging Act or PPPA. The FD&C act deals with misbranding and adulteration of a drug; HIPPA deals with patient confidentiality; and OSHA deals with safety in the work environment.

45. c. The approximate measure of 1 oz is 30 ml; therefore, 6 oz would equal 180 ml.

46. d. The sig code indicates, "Take one to two tablets four times a day as needed for pain."

47. a. Use ratio and proportion. Setup: 40 mEq/1,000 ml = x mEq/60 ml; x = 2.4 mEq.

48. a. The laminar flow hood should be inspected at least every six months.

49. b. H2 blockers work by inhibiting acid secretion in the parietal cells of the stomach and are used in the treatment of GERD.

50. d. Using the allegation chart, the parts are 5:5 which equals 1:1.

51. c. A five-micron filter is sufficient to filter any glass fragments out of the solution. When removing medication from an ampule, you must use either a filter needle or filter straw.

52. b. OBRA was originally intended for Medicaid patients, but many states have adopted the requirement of pharmacists counseling patients for any new prescription order received.

53. d. Both PTCB and ICPT require that once nationally certified, by either organization, a pharmacy technician must complete a minimum of 20 hours of continuing education, including 1 hour of pharmacy law every two years for recertification purposes.

54. c. For accuracy purposes, you would use the syringe that is closest to the dose needed, but more than the dose needed. The 10 ml syringe would be okay to use, but would have less accuracy than the 5 ml syringe.

55. b. Use ratio and proportion. Setup: 5 mg/2.2 lb = x mg/142 lb; x = 322.7 mg.

56. c. *Antitussive* refers to medication used for a cough. The respiratory system would be the organ system associated with cough.

57. d. Use ratio and proportion. Setup: 0.07 kg/100 ml = x kg/400 ml; x = 0.28 kg.

58. b. Use ratio and proportion. Setup: 125 mg/5 ml = x mg/360 ml; x = 9,000 mg. New setup: 500 mg/tablet = 9,000 mg/x tablets; x = 18 tablets.

59. c. Use ratio and proportion. Setup: 2 g/100 g = 1 g/x g; x g = 50 g.

60. d. Room temperature should be 15 to 30 degrees Celsius, which is 59 to 86 degrees Fahrenheit.

61. c. Zolpidem or Ambien® is a schedule IV controlled substance. Schedule IV drugs are generally anti-anxiety drugs such as benzodiazepines or drugs used for sleep.

62. b. A formulary is the list of drugs that a pharmacy makes available for a physician to prescribe. You also will see the term *formulary* indicating what drugs insurance companies will cover.

63. c. "Take one teaspoon after meals" is indicated as "1 tsp pc prn." You need to be wary, as the term *ac* means the drug should be taken before meals, and *pc* means the drug should be taken after meals.

64. b. Any protocol established can be found in the pharmacy procedures manual located in the pharmacy setting.

65. c. Intravenous piggybacks, or IVPB, are small-volume IVs used in the administration of drugs. Generally, the volume is between 50 to 250 ml, and the flow rate is 30 to 60 minutes to deliver the drug required.

66. b. The proper cleaning method for the laminar flow hood is side-to-side motions from the back of the hood to the front of the hood away from the HEPA filter with a clean cloth. The solution used to clean it is usually isopropyl alcohol 70%.

67. b. Use ratio and proportion. Setup: 80 ml/1h = x ml/24 hrs = 1,920 ml = 2 L bags.

68. d. Use ratio and proportion. Setup: 250 mg/5 ml = 400 mg/x ml; x = 8 ml.

69. d. Insert your answer from problem 68 into your directions and multiply: (8 ml)(3)(10) = 240 ml.

70. c. Alprazolam, which is the same as Xanax®, is in the class of drug called benzodiazepines. Zolpidem is what is known as a non-benzodiazepine. Metoprolol is a beta-blocker, and azithromycin is a macrolide antibiotic.

71. c. The pricing of prescription is cost plus the markup of 30%. This can easily be solved by first finding what the percent markup is. To find the percent, simply enter 5.75 and multiply this by 30 in your calculator. Then hit the percent key. $1.73; $5.75 + $1.73 = $7.48.

72. b. 5 ml = 1 teaspoon and 15 ml = 1 tablespoon. Setup: 5 ml/1 tsp = 15 ml/x tsp; x = 3 tsp.

73. c. The first two days require 24 tabs, the next two days require 16 tabs, and the next two days require four tabs: (24) + (16) + (4) = 44 tabs.

74. a. According to USP 797, it is recommended that all compounding in the laminar airflow hood be done at least six inches inside the hood.

75. c. The form used to order CII drugs is a DEA Form 222.

76. d. A mlodipine is a calcium channel blocker, nitroglycerin is a vasodilator, enalapril is an ACE inhibitor, and atenolol is a beta-blocker.

77. a. BC3421234 is invalid. (3) + (2) + (2) = 7; (4) + (1) + (3) = 8; (8)(2) = 16; (16) + (7) = 23.

78. c. A diuretic regulates the fluid level in the body by increasing the urine output from the kidneys, anti-inflammatories treat inflammation, antipyretics treat fever, and benzodiazepines treat anxiety.

79. d. *The Orange Book* is used to identify generic equivalence.

80. b. A 0.22 to 0.3 microns filter is considered to be sufficient for a sterilizing filter. The rationale is that 0.22 microns will take out any bacteria but will not remove viruses (which are much smaller).

81. d. Use ratio and proportion. Setup: 1,000 mg/1,000 ml = x mg/10 ml; x = 10 mg.

82. c. Any decision requiring professional judgment should be done by a pharmacist. The use of over-the-counter decongestants can cause problems in patients with heart disease or diabetes.

83. d. Vicodin® is the same as hydrocodone with acetaminophen, and it is a CIII drug. Acetaminophen with codeine is the same as Tylenol® No. tabs (*example:* Tylenol® No. 3), which are also CIII drugs. Oxycodone with acetaminophen is the same as Percocet®, which is a CII drug.

84. a. Use ratio and proportion. Setup: 1 tab/300 mg = x tabs/1,200 mg; x = 4 tabs.

85. a. The IV piggyback is a small bag attached to the main line IV, which will administer medication over a flow rate of around 30 to 60 minutes. IV push or bolus is the administration of a drug over a short period of time via a syringe/needle in an IV line, and it is usually indicated for emergency type medications.

86. b. Use ratio and proportion. Setup: 1 g/50 ml = x g/200 ml; x = 4 g. New setup: 4 g/500 ml = x g/100 ml; x = 0.8 g. 0.8/100 ml is the definition of 0.8%.

87. a. *Facts and Comparisons* is the most updated reference book, as it comes in a three-ring binder that is updated monthly with inserts mailed to the pharmacy for removal and replacement. Generally, updating this manual is one of the tasks for the pharmacy technician.

88. b. Use ratio and proportion. Setup: 1 g/100 g = x g/60 g; x = 0.6 g.

89. b. The patient will use 75 units daily for 30 days, which equals 2,250 units. Since a vial of insulin contains 1,000 units (1 ml = 100 units and 1 vial is 10 ml), three vials must be dispensed.

90. b. Robitussin DM® is guaifenesin with dextromethorphan. The other drugs indicated are formulated to be long-acting or sustained-release.

Diagnostic Test Score: _____ of 100 questions right

One of the main reasons you took this practice diagnostic test is to see where your strengths and weaknesses lie. Reviewing the material (and answering the practice questions) in Chapters 4–12 should improve your score significantly. Make a note of what you need to review and allot your remaining study time accordingly.

Success is the result of good planning and hard work.

4 ▶ Prescriptions and Abbreviations

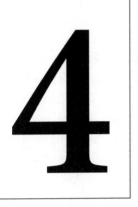

CHAPTER OVERVIEW

In the retail pharmacy setting, the legal form a physician must fill out to be filled at a licensed pharmacy setting is what we call a prescription. Prescriptions must be correct and verified, and they have specific rules which govern filling and refilling them. This chapter will cover the different aspects of a prescription, as well as the abbreviations which are vital for the pharmacy technician to understand in both reading the prescription, medication, or IV admixture orders and solving certain types of calculations in the process.

KEY TERMS

prescription
policy and procedures manual
controlled drugs
abbreviations
DAW

auxiliary label
"Rx Only"
NDC number
references

The Prescription

A **prescription** is a lawful order for a specific medication, to be filled at a licensed pharmacy. This order is generally written by a licensed physician—but depending on individual state laws, it can also be written by other health professionals (with restrictions), such as dentists, veterinarians, physician assistants, and pharmacists. Prescriptions can be hand delivered or sent by fax, computer, or phone. All handed in or faxed prescription orders must have the physician's signature. If the physician is unable to call in a prescription order, a representative of the physician, such as a nurse, may call in the prescription order. Federal law mandates that only pharmacists may receive phoned-in prescription orders.

The role of the pharmacy technician in accepting prescription orders by a customer begins with understanding the proper procedures involved. Procedures are generally stated in the pharmacy **policy and procedures manual** and should be reviewed in the beginning of one's employment in a particular pharmacy setting.

Written Parts of the Prescription

Every prescription order received should contain the following information:

- prescriber's name, address, phone number
- name of the patient for whom the prescription was written
- date the prescription was written
- the medication ordered, including name, strength, dosage form, and quantity
- directions for use
- number of refills permitted
- whether a generic drug is permitted to replace a brand-name drug (if not, the prescription will say **DAW**, or dispense as written)
- prescriber's Drug Enforcement Agency (DEA) number, if this is a controlled medication order
- physician's signature

Here's an example of a completed prescription:

Dr. Irene Cortiz-Colella
366 Holly Lane, Denver, CO 80219 (303) 111-1111

Patient ___Joe Medina_____ Date ___November 3, 2010_____

Address ___560 Benzodiazepine Avenue_____

Rx Zoloft 100 mg #60

Sig: i po qd x 60 days for depression

___Dr. Irene Cortiz-Colella___ M.D.

DAW: ____ Refills __6__ DEA REG. No. _____

Prescription Refills

The refilling of an individual prescription is up to the physician writing the order, but there are some legal guidelines that must be met depending on if the drug is a controlled substance or not.

The Controlled Substances Act (CSA), reviewed in Chapter 5, lists **controlled drugs** into five classes, or schedules. Schedule I substances have the highest abuse potential, while schedule V have the least. Under this law, refill of a prescription and how long it is good for once written is dependent on its schedule or if it is a noncontrolled drug that is not considered to have an abuse potential:

- If a prescription is a controlled drug according to schedule II of the Controlled Substances Act, the prescription cannot be refilled—regardless of whether the physician requests a refill.
- If a prescription is a controlled drug and found in schedule III through schedule V, the prescription may have up to five refills maximum. The prescription is also valid for six months from the date of issue.
- If a prescription is a noncontrolled drug, the prescription may have up to 11 refills maximum. The prescription is also valid for 12 months from the date of issue.

Prescription Validity

One role of the pharmacy technician is to ensure a prescription is legal and valid, and not a forgery. In the retail setting, this problem does arise and can frequently be difficult to spot. Forgeries can be as simple as replacing a quantity or as complex as writing a false prescription entirely.

Passed in April of 2008, the Tamper Resistant Prescription Act was a federal law requiring Medicaid physicians to write their prescriptions on prescription pads that are easily recognized as legitimate. *All* Medicaid prescriptions must be written on tamper-resistant prescription pads in order to be eligible for pharmacy reimbursement. These pads are made of paper that makes it more difficult to copy completed or blank individual prescriptions and to erase or modify information on a prescription.

Another way to help prevent fraud is to know how to interpret a verifiable Drug Enforcement Agency number on each controlled prescription ordered. If a DEA number is incorrect, this could be indicative of a fake prescription. The Controlled Substance Act also indicates the need for a physician to have a DEA number to write a prescription for any controlled substance. The DEA number consists of two letters. The first letter will either be an A or B and the second letter will be the first letter of the physician's last name followed by seven numbers. The pharmacy technician can easily identify a correct DEA number by following the below steps:

Correct DEA Number?

First letter will always be A or B.

Second letter will always be the first letter of the physicians last name.

A mathematical calculation exists which ensures that the DEA number is correct:

- Add the first, third, and fifth numbers to get your first answer.
- Add the second, fourth, and sixth numbers, then multiply your total by two to get your second answer.
- Add your first answer with your second answer. The last digit of this sum will be the same as the last digit of the DEA number.

Example: Dr. Hodson DEA No: AH123456<u>3</u>

1) $1 + 3 + 5 = 9$

2) $2 + 4 + 6 = 12 \times 2 = 24$

3) $9 + 24 = 3\underline{3}$ ⟶ AH123456<u>3</u>

Prescription Interpretation

Understanding a written prescription order is essential. This allows the pharmacy technician to put the necessary (and correct) information into the computer.

Upon receipt of a prescription, the pharmacy technician should be able to interpret the prescription fully and notice any missing information that may be necessary to fill the prescription order properly. The pharmacy technician can complete some missing information, but the pharmacist must add any missing information that requires professional judgment.

Prescription Directions

In most cases, the directions (*sig* means "take thou") are written in shorthand, or an abbreviated form, that allows directions to be written easily. Directions generally include how and when to take the medication ordered.

The pharmacy technician should have knowledge of the abbreviations in prescription orders. This is the only way a pharmacy technician will be able to correctly input directions into the computer and ensure the correct directions will be on the pharmacy label when the medication is dispensed.

Below is the list of **abbreviations** you should know not only for the national exam, but when working in the pharmacy setting as well:

Commonly Used Abbreviations

ac	before meals
ad	right ear
am	morning
as	left ear
ASAP	as soon as possible
au	both ears
bid	twice a day
c	with
cc	cubic centimeter (same as ml or milliliter)

d	day
DAW	dispense as written
dc	discontinue
gtt	drop
h	hour
hs	at bedtime
i	one
ii	two
iii	three
iv	four
od	right eye
opth	ophthalmic (for the eye)
os	left eye
otic	for the ear
ou	each eye
nte	not to exceed
p	after
pc	after meals
pm	evening
po	by mouth
pr	In rectum
prn	as needed
pv	in vagina
q	every
qd	every day or daily
q4h	every four hours
qid	four times a day
qod	every other day
qs	quantity sufficient or to make
qsad	add quantity to make specific volume
s	without
ss	one-half
sig	directions
sl	under the tongue
stat	at once or now
supp	suppository
tid	three times a day
ud	as directed

From the list of abbreviations, we are able to create sentences to give directions.

> **Example:** *ii gtts ou qid ud*
> **Translation:** Place two drops into each eye, four times a day as directed.

Prescription Misinterpretation

Human error can lead to misinterpretation of prescriptions sometimes. This is especially true with the names of medications and the prescribing directions. To avoid problems, an understanding of abbreviations is vital for the pharmacy technician, as is conveying these directions in an easy-to-understand format, so that patients understand completely how they are required to take the medication. Never assume that directions can be understood easily by a customer or patient. You need to make the directions as simple and easy to understand as possible when putting directions into the computer.

> **Example:** *1 tab po bid x 10 days*
> **Translation:** Take one tablet orally twice a day for ten days.

Now let's make it easier to understand for the customer:

> **Example:** *1 tab po bid x 10 days*
> **Translation:** Take one tablet **by mouth** two times a day for ten days.

Another example:

> **Example:** *1 pr qd prn*
> **Translation:** Insert one rectally daily as needed.

Now let's make it easier to understand for the customer:

> **Remove foil and** insert 1 **suppository in rectum once a day** as needed.

In some cases, the prescription directions may be difficult to interpret. If there's any question as far as the validity of information on a prescription, the pharmacist should be notified. In most cases, the pharmacist will be able to correct the issue or, if necessary, call the physician for clarification.

The medication information itself is as vital as the directions for the medication's use. The correct interpretation of the prescription, including strength and quantity, is important. Misinterpretation does occur, involving thousands of drugs, because of poor physician handwriting and drug names that sound the same phonetically. An understanding of trade and generic drug names is necessary to interpret a prescription order correctly.

If a prescription order indicates *DAW*, this means dispense as written, and indicates that the physician writing the prescription order wants exactly the medication written on the order. That does not mean the customer cannot ask the pharmacist to contact the physician to change the medication, as the customer's insurance company may not cover the exact drug on the prescription in some cases.

Prescription Transfer

Federal law states only a pharmacist can accept a prescription transferred from one pharmacy to another. State laws differ as to whether the original prescription is cancelled when a transfer is made. Federal law mandates that all prescription transfers must be handwritten on a new prescription form (hard copy) by the pharmacist receiving the transfer, with other essential information. Some pharmacies, such as Walgreens, have a database of all prescriptions filled by Walgreens within the United States, which makes prescriptions easy to transfer within the chain of pharmacies.

The Prescription Label

Finished prescription labels derived from the computer should contain the following information:

- pharmacy name, address, and telephone number
- prescription or serial number
- patient's name
- dispensing date
- medication name, strength, dosage form, and quantity
- directions for use
- prescriber's name
- expiration date
- number of refills allowed
- necessary **auxiliary labels**, including: **"Rx Only"**
- **National Drug Code (NDC) number**

Sample Prescription label

Norma's Rx
1524 South Euphoria Lane
Denver, CO 80054
000-305-9988

Rx 116039430   11/03/2010 jm
Joe Medina   Dr. Irene Cortiz-Colella

Take 1 tablet by mouth twice a day for depression.

Zoloft (Sertraline HCl) 100 mg #60
NDC No. 0049-4960-50

Refills left: 4
Rx exp: 11/3/2011

Some states differ as to whether both the trade name and generic name must appear on the prescription label, as well as the expiration date and number of refills. For federal purposes, all of the information in the prescription label above should be included.

What Is an NDC Number?

The NDC number is the National Drug Code number which should appear on every prescription bottle as well as the "Rx Only" label. The number is similar to our Social Security Number (SSN) in that it identifies the product in the container. It comes in three sets of digits of which each set has its own meaning.

Example: **00000–0000–00**

1st set of digits indicates the manufacturer.
2nd set of digits indicates the drug product.
3rd set of digits indicates the package size.

Auxiliary Labels

Auxiliary labels are used to provide additional general information about the proper use of a drug that is not included in the directions. Generally, they are color-coded, and the computer will ensure the correct auxiliary label is placed on the prescription label, so there's no need for the pharmacy technician to memorize which auxiliary labels go with which medication.

May cause drowsiness
Avoid sunlight
For the Eye
"Rx Only"

The "Rx Only" label replaces the old label, which said, "Federal law prohibits dispensing without a prescription," per the FDA Modernization Act of 1997.

Pharmacy Drug Recalls

FDA drug recalls occur from time to time, if a manufactured legend (prescription) drug product appears to have serious problems associated with it. Drug recalls are given in three different classes which indicate the severity of the recall:

- Class I recall: A situation in which there is a reasonable probability that the use of or exposure will cause serious adverse health consequences or death
- Class II recall: A situation in which use of or exposure may cause temporary or medically reversible adverse health consequences; or where the probability of serious adverse health consequences is remote
- Class III recall: A situation in which use of or exposure is not likely to cause adverse health consequences

Reference Books Found in the Pharmacy Setting

The pharmacy should have **reference** books that allow a health professional, including the pharmacy technician, to look up specific information as needed. Below is a chart of the most common reference sources found in the pharmacy setting, and what kinds of information are offered in each.

REFERENCE	INFORMATION PROVIDED	OTHER USEFUL INFORMATION
United States Pharmacopeia	drug standards	required in the pharmacy setting
USP—Drug Information or USP-DI		
Volume I	information for the health professional	
Volume II	advice for the patient	written in easy-to-understand language
Volume III	approved drug products and legal requirements	
Remington's Pharmaceutical	information for compounding purposes	contains physical characteristics of different drugs and recipes
Facts and Comparisons	drug information	easy to read; is the most updated reference source; is the most used drug information reference for pharmacists
Physician's Desk Reference or PDR	information about drugs, mainly inserts from drug manufacturers	limited information, as the book is dependent on which drug inserts are included; difficult to read
American Drug Index	brief information about all trade and generic drugs available	if more information needed, go to the Facts and Comparisons

REFERENCE	INFORMATION PROVIDED	OTHER USEFUL INFORMATION
Handbook of Over-the-Counter Drugs	information on all OTC drugs on the market	includes not only active drugs, but also inactive ingredients
Handbook of Injectable Drugs	information about IV solutions and drug-drug compatibilities	includes charts that indicate compatibility of drugs and IV solutions
Redbook	information concerning the average wholesale pricing of prescriptions	for insurance or third-party pricing
The Orange Book	listing of generic drug equivalencies compared to other generic drugs or trade name drugs	used to help in the ordering of generic drugs

Drug Expiration Date

A drug's *expiration date* is the time frame for which a drug is "good," according to the manufacturer. Generally, the actual expiration date can be further out than the date given, but because there is little scientific proof to support this, drug companies will set an earlier expiration date.

The expiration date of a product will most times be by month and year. The actual expiration date, though, is the last day of the month and year indicated.

Example: A 12/2010 expiration date on the bottle really means 12/31/2010 is the actual expiration date.

To ensure products do not expire while in the pharmacy setting, it is important to rotate stock accordingly by placing drugs that are to expire sooner in front of drugs that are to expire later. This can easily be done when replenishing medications on a daily basis.

Practice Questions

1. Interpret the following directions:

   i cap po qid × 10d

   a. Take one capsule by mouth four times a day for ten days.
   b. Take one capsule by mouth three times a day for ten days.
   c. Take one capsule by mouth twice a day for ten days.
   d. Take one capsule by mouth once a day for ten days.

2. Interpret the following directions:

   ii tab po tid × 7d.

   a. Take two tablets by mouth four times a day for seven days.
   b. Take two tablets by mouth three times a day for seven days.
   c. Take two tablets by mouth twice a day for seven days.
   d. Take two tablets by mouth once a day for seven days.

3. Interpret the following directions:

   i pr hs

   a. Take one as needed at bedtime.
   b. Insert one in rectum before bedtime.
   c. Insert one in rectum at bedtime.
   d. Insert one in rectum after bedtime.

4. How many tablets need to be dispensed for the following directions:

   sig: vi tab po tid × 2d; iv po bid × 2d; iii po qd × 2d; i po qd × 2d then dc

   a. 28 tablets
   b. 36 tablets
   c. 48 tablets
   d. 60 tablets

Using the following information to answer questions 5 and 6:

   Percocet® #30
   sig: i – ii po qid ud prn pain

5. Interpret the above directions.
   a. Take one by mouth as needed for pain.
   b. Take one to two by mouth as needed for pain.
   c. Take one to two by mouth four times a day as needed for pain.
   d. Take one to two by mouth four times a day as directed as needed for pain.

6. If Percocet® is a schedule II drug, what is the maximum number of refills allowed for this prescription?
   a. 0
   b. 1
   c. 5
   d. 11

7. Of the following drug recalls, which one is the most serious, indicating that a patient may be harmed?
   a. class I
   b. class II
   c. class III
   d. class IV

8. Of the following reference sources, which one deals with the term *incompatibility*?
   a. *Facts and Comparisons*
   b. *PDR*
   c. *Handbook of Injectable Drugs*
   d. *Remington's Pharmaceutical Sciences*

9. Of the following reference sources, which one involves manufacturer drug inserts?
  a. *Facts and Comparisons*
  b. *PDR*
  c. *Handbook of Injectable Drugs*
  d. *Remington's Pharmaceutical Sciences*

10. Based on the following directions, which Cortisporin® drops are you going to use?

sig: ii gtts ou bid × 10d

  a. Cortisporin® Otic drops
  b. Cortisporin® Ophthalmic drops
  c. Both drops can be used.
  d. The directions have nothing to do with drops.

11. What does the third set of numbers refer to when we are talking about the NDC number?
  a. the manufacturer
  b. the product
  c. the package size
  d. the classification of drug

12. What does DAW mean?
  a. to fill a prescription for quantity asked for
  b. to fill a prescription for drug asked for
  c. The prescription order must be delivered.
  d. It is allowable to substitute a generic version of this drug.

Using the following information, answer questions 13, 14, and 15:

amoxicillin 150 mg 11/03/2010
sig: i po tid × 10d
Dr. Irene Ortiz
Refills _____ DAW __

13. How many capsules are needed to fill this prescription order?
  a. 10 capsules
  b. 20 capsules
  c. 30 capsules
  d. 40 capsules

14. What is the maximum number of refills this prescription can have, with doctor approval?
  a. 0
  b. 1
  c. 5
  d. 11

15. How long is this prescription valid to be filled at a licensed pharmacy?
  a. ten days
  b. three months
  c. six months
  d. one year

16. What would the true expiration date be for a drug that has 04/2012 as the expiration date imprinted on the manufacturer's container?
  a. 3/31/2012
  b. 4/01/2012
  c. 4/30/2012
  d. 5/01/2012

17. Interpret the following directions:

ii po q12h pc prn indigestion.

  a. Take two by mouth every 12 hours as needed.
  b. Take two by mouth every 12 hours as needed for indigestion.
  c. Take two by mouth every 12 hours before meals as needed for indigestion.
  d. Take two by mouth every 12 hours after meals as needed for indigestion.

18. If one teaspoonful (tsp) is equal to 5 ml in volume, what is the total volume needed to fill this prescription or last the full 30 days?

sig: 1/2 tsp po bid × 30d

  a. 50 ml
  b. 100 ml
  c. 150 ml
  d. 200 ml

19. Which of the following is a false statement?
  a. Being human causes misinterpretation of prescriptions sometimes.
  b. The medication being prescribed is as vital as the directions for the medication's use.
  c. Always assume directions can be easily understood by a customer or patient.
  d. If a prescription order indicates DAW, this means it should be dispensed as written.

20. Which of the following is most likely to be a correct DEA number for a Dr. Robert Plick?
  a. AR4637810
  b. AR4637816
  c. AP4637810
  d. BP4637813

Answers and Explanations

1. a. Take one capsule by mouth four times a day for ten days. Remember: *qd* is once a day, *bid* is twice a day, *tid* is three times a day and *qid* is four times a day.

2. b. Take two tablets by mouth three times a day for seven days.

3. c. Insert one in rectum at bedtime. *Hs* means always at bedtime and not before or after. *Pr* means "pertaining to the rectum," but for easy to understand directions, "in rectum" would apply.

4. d. The total is 60 tabs. If we break it down in days: on day one, we would dispense 18 tabs; on day two, 18 tabs; on day three, eight tabs; on day four, eight tabs; on day five, three tabs; on day six, three tabs; on day seven, one tab; and on day eight, one tab. If we add these tabs up, it would come to 60 tablets total.

5. d. Take one to two by mouth four times a day as directed, as needed for pain.

6. a. The maximum number of refills for a CII drug is 0; for schedule III to V, it is 5 refills; for noncontrolled drugs, the maximum refill amount would be 11.

7. a. A class I drug recall would be the most serious, meaning it may cause harm to a patient. class II is less serious, as harm to patient is remotely possible, but highly unlikely. In class II, there is no harm expected for the patient, as the product does not meet FDA guidelines.

8. c. *Handbook of Injectable Drugs* is used to look for compatibility or incompatibility of injectable drugs or solutions. *Facts and Comparisons* is a reference source for drug therapy, as is the *PDR*. *Remington's Pharmaceutical Sciences* is a book that deals with questions involving compounding.

9. b. The *PDR* is a source for drug information but is limited as it contains only drug inserts from drug manufacturers.

10. b. The directions imply that the drops are to be placed in each eye, so you would use the ophthalmic drops—the otic drops would be for the ear.

11. c. The third set of digits of the NDC number is the package size. The first set would be the manufacturer, and the second set of digits would identify the product itself.

12. b. DAW, or dispense as written, specifically asks the pharmacy to fill the medication as prescribed or ordered. A change can be made only if the pharmacist were to get approval from the physician to do so.

13. c. The directions "one capsule by mouth three times a day for ten days" will tell you how many capsules you need if you simply follow the directions and multiply: (1 cap) (3 days) (10 days) = 30 capsules. Although we have yet to go over calculations, this tells you the importance of understanding abbreviations. You need to know how to figure this one out on your own.

14. d. The maximum number of refills would be 11, as amoxicillin is a noncontrolled drug. Although we have not reviewed specific drugs yet, you should have figured out an antibiotic would not be controlled or have a potential for abuse.

15. d. Since this drug is noncontrolled, the prescription is good for one year. The maximum number of refills for a CII drug is 0. Schedule III to V drugs have 5 refills. And for noncontrolled drugs, the maximum refill amount would be 11.

16. c. The true expiration date given on a manufacturer's container, when written in the month/year format, is always the last day of the month in the year shown. In this case, that's 4/30/2012.

17. d. Take two by mouth every 12 hours after meals as needed for indigestion.

18. c. The directions imply what the total volume will be if we insert our volume and multiply. In this case, you are told that 1 tsp is equal to 5 ml. If this is the case, then 0.5 tsp would be equal to 2.5 ml, or one-half of 5 ml. To solve: (2.5 ml)(3 times a day)(10 days) = 150 ml.

19. c. You should *never* assume that directions can be understood easily by the customer or patient. That would be one reason that counseling customers/patients is so important.

20. d. The first letter of a DEA number is either A or B, and the second letter is the first letter of the physician's last name. The mathematical steps involve adding the first, third and fifth set of digits to get a total, then add the second, fourth and sixth set of digits to get a total, which you will multiply by 2. Then simply add your two totals, and the last number of your new total is the last digit of the DEA number.

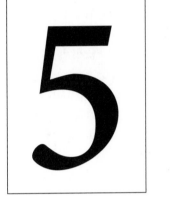

5 ▶ Pharmacy Law

CHAPTER OVERVIEW

The practice of pharmacology is one of the most heavily regulated professions in the United States. Although a basic understanding of pharmacology is the center of a technician's education, knowledge of both state and federal law is required to practice effectively in this profession. This chapter will help you understand the concepts of some of the more important laws that may appear on the national exams, which, more importantly, you will need to understand when working in the pharmacy. Most common pharmacy reference books will also be discussed.

KEY TERMS

adulteration	law
board of pharmacy (BOP)	legend drug
case law	legislative law
code of ethics	MedWatch
common law	misbranding
contract law	National Association of the Boards of Pharmacy
criminal law	protected health information (PHI)
Drug Enforcement Administration (DEA)	orphan drug
ethics	state board of pharmacy
Food and Drug Administration (FDA)	

The need to understand the specific **laws** governing the pharmacy profession cannot be overstated. There are situations in which a pharmacy technician will make a decision that involves a law in some respect. As mentioned in Chapter 2, there are state and federal laws which the technician needs to understand. Since states do differ, we will simply discuss federal law on which the national exam is based. Be sure to check with the pharmacy board of your own state to learn more about the state laws that will affect your job. Finally, it is necessary for you to understand that due to changing roles, where pharmacy technicians are essentially taking over the dispensing functions once reserved for pharmacists, a pharmacy technician can be held accountable and liable for a medication error in a court of law.

Introduction to Law

Laws are the principles and regulations established in a community by a governing body and applicable to its people, whether in the form of legislation or policies recognized and enforced by judicial decision. Laws also provide resolution to conflicts between two parties. In pharmacy, the goal is to protect the health and welfare of the patients, while also protecting the practitioners from individuals who would defraud a pharmacy to obtain medication. Laws must evolve to meet the changes or challenges that are presented in the community.

The Sources of Laws

Laws are developed from a multitude of sources in an effort to best reflect the needs of the people they serve. In the United States, the core of our laws comes from the Constitution. U.S. laws are broken down into four types. First is constitutional law, which is drawn from the Constitution and the Bill of Rights. Next is **legislative law**, which is drawn from the legislative branch of the government (U.S. Congress and state legislatures). Third is administrative law, which is derived from the executive branch of the government (the president or state governor and their cabinets). Last is **common law**, also known as **case law**, which is drawn from the judicial branch of the government (the court system). Collectively, these laws govern all aspects of the practice of pharmacy.

Divisions of Law

The legal system in the United States is divided into three categories. **Criminal law** is enforced by a state representative against persons or companies. In civil law, a plaintiff will bring a suit against an alleged defendant. **Contract law** pertains to an agreement between two or more parties and is typically enforced in civil court.

Criminal Law

Criminal laws pertain to violations of criminal statutes and codes. Punishments for these crimes include monetary fines, imprisonment, or death in certain cases. These punishments are separated into two categories: misdemeanors and felonies. Misdemeanors are lesser crimes that are punishable by fines and/or imprisonment of less than one year. Felonies, on the other hand, are punishable by larger fines and imprisonment of more than one year. In many states, a felony conviction is grounds for revocation of a license to practice medicine. As a pharmacy provider, termination of employment and possible prosecution under criminal law can occur if the technician participates in drug diversion (stealing), prescription forgery, or theft.

Civil Law

Civil wrongdoings are often referred to as *torts*. A tort is an injury, either physical or nonphysical, that is inflicted on one person by another. The person who caused the injury is legally responsible for their actions. Although the injury may be unintentional, the guilty party is still liable. These injuries include assault, battery, fraud, libel, negligence, slander, theft, and even wrongful death. Most civil law cases against healthcare professionals are for malpractice, which is professional misconduct or negligence—the failure to exercise reasonable care. These penalties are almost always monetary, in an effort to rectify the damage inflicted on the plaintiff. In pharmacy, a technician can be sued by a patient if it is found that the technician has either performed a duty outside the scope of his or her practice or acted negligently, which resulted in the injury or death of a patient.

Contract Law

Contract law deals with agreements between two or more parties. A contract is a legally binding exchange which requires the involved parties to do or not do certain things. If any party fails to uphold the terms of the contract, legal action may be taken. In most cases, it is a civil matter and is resolved by monetary means. In some pharmacies, the employment contract states that the employer will pay for technicians to continue their education. In return, the contract may require the employee to work for the employer for a specified amount of time. Additional instances of contract law in pharmacy include agreements between pharmacy providers and insurance companies, specifying the terms of payment for claims. If either party does not adhere to the terms of the agreement, the other party may ask for the money in the agreement to be returned.

State and Federal Law

State and federal courts are not necessarily independent of each other. Many state and federal laws interact, creating overlap between the courts. The difference is that federal courts handle cases that violate the laws that Congress has enacted. States have the authority to enact laws in areas where Congress has already acted, assuming the laws do not conflict with the federal versions. The federal law will always supersede the state, unless the state law is stricter than the federal version. In these cases, the state law will prevail. An example is the classification of Valium. According to the **Drug Enforcement Administration** (DEA), Valium is a class IV controlled substance; but in the state of New York, it is treated as a class II and is

considered to have a greater potential for abuse. More recently, marijuana has been considered to have no medicinal value by federal law, but today we are seeing medicinal marijuana dispensaries opening up in some states (with highly restrictive regulation).

Ethics

In the workplace, **ethics** are a system of moral values given to a vocation or profession to follow. As a pharmacy technician, it is imperative that you follow the ethical standards of pharmacy practice. It is important to remember that professional behavior and moral character are just as important in pharmacy as knowledge of medications.

Pharmacy Technician Code of Ethics

The American Association of pharmacy technicians (AAPT) has its own **code of ethics** for its membership. These ethics guide the technician in relationships with patients, healthcare professionals, and society. The principles of the pharmacy technician code of ethics include the following:

- A pharmacy technician's first consideration is to ensure the health and safety of the patient and to use knowledge and skills to the best of his/her ability in serving patients.
- A pharmacy technician supports and promotes honesty and integrity in the profession, which includes a duty to observe the law, maintain the highest moral and ethical conduct at all times, and uphold the ethical principles of the profession.
- A pharmacy technician assists and supports the pharmacists in the safe, efficacious, and cost-effective distribution of health services and healthcare resources.
- A pharmacy technician respects and values the abilities of pharmacists, colleagues, and other healthcare professionals.

- A pharmacy technician maintains competency in his/her practice and continually enhances his/her professional knowledge and expertise.
- A pharmacy technician respects and supports the patient's individuality, dignity, and confidentiality.
- A pharmacy technician respects the confidentiality of a patient's records and discloses pertinent information only with proper authorization.
- A pharmacy technician never assists in dispensing, promoting, or distributing medication or medical devices that are not of good quality or do not meet the standards required by law.
- A pharmacy technician does not engage in any activity that will discredit the profession, and will expose, without fear or favor, illegal or unethical conduct.
- A pharmacy technician associates with and engages in the support of organizations that promote the profession of pharmacy through the utilization and enhancement of pharmacy technicians.

Making Ethical Decisions

To practice as an effective pharmacy technician, one must have a strong knowledge of ethical issues that may relate to the profession. In addition, technicians must balance their personal value system with their professional practice. What an individual has experienced in his or her life will come into play when making ethical decisions. These decisions will arise each day and have consequences for all parties involved. The following steps will help the pharmacy technician to better assess the decision-making process so that the appropriate action can be taken.

Identify the Problem

The first step in making a good ethical decision is to identify the problem. In many cases, there can be multiple problems which have led to the current situation. It is important to be able to identify the core issue and work to resolve that first, as it can lead to a resolution for all related issues.

Gather Data

Before any decision can be made, information should be gathered in an effort to make the most informed decision possible. The most effective way to obtain this information is to ask questions, review documentation, and research the situation in question. This will help to provide the technician with the most complete picture of the situation. This also ensures that the correct ethical route is identified.

Analyze Data

The most effective way to come to an ethical conclusion is to analyze the data. When making a decision, all parties involved must be considered, with a focus on the consequences for the potential actions. Many times, all alternative solutions will need to be explored prior to making a final decision.

Create an Action Plan

After all the information has been reviewed, a decision must be made about the situation. The action plan should be made based on the decision, as the technician begins to solve the issue in question. This plan should include measurable steps toward an outcome. If handled properly, the plan will be as accommodating as possible to both sides, while remaining unbiased, and resolve the issue.

Assess the Results

After the resolution of the issue, the final step is to evaluate the results from the action plan. This helps to ensure that the correct decision was made and that all parties involved are adhering to the plan. It also makes future situations easier to address and handle.

Federal Laws

Federal pharmacy laws are the core of the industry. In many instances, these are the laws that set the standards for the practice of pharmacy. They pertain to the safety of the general public. Although there are state laws that overlap or even supersede the federal ones, the minimum standard for safety is held in place by the federal laws. In addition, there are regulatory bodies that enforce these laws. The body that deals directly with the manufacture and review of the medications is the **Food and Drug Administration** (FDA). Most laws found in the following section are governed by this body, whose laws have shaped the pharmaceutical industry in the United States. Although the background on the following laws will include dates to indicate when the laws were passed, there will be no dates tested on the national exams.

Pure Food and Drug Act

Enacted in 1906, the Pure Food and Drug Act prohibited the interstate distribution or sale of adulterated (made less pure) or misbranded (improperly labeled) food or drugs. It was aimed primarily at the meat-packing industry after Upton Sinclair's novel exposé *The Jungle*, as well as at the patent medicine business. It was the first federal law regulating drugs, and although it was replaced by the Food, Drug, and Cosmetic Act (FD&C Act), it paved the way for the modern FDA.

Food, Drug, and Cosmetic Act

The FD&C Act was enacted in 1938 after the sulfanilamide disaster of the previous year that killed more than 100 patients when Massengill company used diethylene glycol (antifreeze) as a sweetener for an elixir. The law required all drug manufacturers to file a New Drug Application (NDA) with the FDA before any drug could be approved or disapproved for the market. The manufacturers also had to ensure the purity, safety, packaging, and strength of a medication. This act gave the FDA the authority to approve or deny NDAs and conduct inspections to ensure compliance with regulations. This act is the basis for today's pharmacy laws. In addition, it requires medications to be labeled with adequate directions for safe use.

The FD&C Act requires the proper labeling or branding of products and also requires that what is inside the container cannot be changed from what it is labeled to be. It involves violation if there is **misbranding** on the label and any **adulteration** of what is inside the container.

Durham-Humphrey Amendment

This 1951 amendment to the FD&C Act was a response to the FDA's internal classification of prescription (**legend drugs**) and nonprescription (OTC) medications. As these classifications were deemed ineffective, Senators Hubert Humphrey and Carl Durham, both pharmacists, supported legislation that established clear criteria for such decisions. It prohibited dispensing legend drugs without a prescription. This arose due to the lack of oversight and education regarding prescription items, leading many pharmacies to unwittingly sell prescription medications over the counter. Nonlegend medications were not restricted for sale. This law was enacted because the FDA could not approve many new medications under the existing law. Each prescription medication would bear the legend "Caution: Federal law prohibits dispensing this medication without a prescription."

Kefauver-Harris Amendment

Enacted in 1963, the Kefauver-Harris Amendment required that all medications, both prescription and nonprescription, be pure, effective, and safe to use on humans. It also placed prescription drug advertising under the supervision of the FDA, along with qualifications for drug investigators. It required manufacturers to register and to allow inspection of their manufacturing sites. This law was established based on a study of ongoing trade practices in the pharmaceutical industry. This included the marketing of worthless and/or potentially lethal medications. This amendment was enacted in the wake of the thalidomide tragedy of the late 1950s, which caused roughly 10,000 to 20,000 birth defects when used by pregnant women.

The Thalidomide Disaster occurred due to the use of the drug thalidomide by pregnant women for morning sickness. It was not until 1962 that the drug was removed from the market because of its teratogenic (unwanted) effects on the newborn, which included flippers for limbs and internal injuries to various organs. By that time, over 20,000 babies were born with the defects associated with this drug, and today we call them the "thalidomide babies."

Controlled Substances Act

The Comprehensive Drug Abuse Prevention and Control Act, also known as the Controlled Substances Act (CSA), was enacted in 1970. It requires the pharmaceutical industry to keep records and maintain security measures for certain medications. It divided controlled substances into five classes, or schedules. Schedule I substances have the highest abuse potential, while schedule V have the least. Under this law, medications can be added or deleted from schedules, as well as changed to a different schedule, based on DEA action. In addition, individuals or companies can petition for a schedule change. The Drug Enforcement Administration is the regulatory agency for anything relating to controlled drugs.

Controlled Substances: The Five Schedules

SCHEDULE OF DRUG	ABOUT THESE DRUGS	EXAMPLES OF DRUGS
schedule I (CI)	drugs having no accepted medical use in the United States, with a high abuse potential	LSD, crack, mescaline, heroin, marijuana*
schedule II (CII)	drugs having an accepted medical use and a high abuse potential, with severe psychic or physical dependence liability	amphetamines, methadone, opium, Percocet®, Ritalin®, Sublimaze (Fentanyl®), cocaine*
schedule III (CIII)	drugs having an accepted medical use and an abuse potential less than those in schedules I and II	combination narcotics such as Tylenol No.3®, Vicodin®
schedule IV (CIV)	drugs having an accepted medical use and an abuse potential less than those listed in schedule III	benzodiazepines such as lorazepam and alprazolam, as well as hypnotics such as zolpidem or Ambien®
schedule V (CV)	drugs having an accepted medical use and an abuse potential less than those listed in schedule IV	Lomotil or cough preps with codeine such as Robitussin AC®

*Marijuana is now used in some states for medicinal purposes. Cocaine is also used in the hospital setting for facial surgery such as rhinoplasty.

The CSA also deals with the ordering of schedule II drugs by using a DEA Form 222. Any other schedule drug from CIII to CIV or noncontrolled legend (prescription) drug does not require any special procedures. As for the labeling of a controlled substance container, it must have a large C imprinted on the container, as well as the schedule under which the drug is classified. *Example:* CIII.

Poison Prevention Packaging Act

Enacted in 1970, the Poison Prevention Packaging Act created standards for child-resistant packaging. It mandates that containers be manufactured to be very difficult for young children to open. It requires that some OTC medications, and nearly all legend drugs, be packaged in child-resistant containers. These containers cannot be opened by 80% of children younger than five years old, but can be opened by 90% of adults.

Medications that are dispensed in hospitals and nursing homes are not typically packaged in child-resistant packages because children do not usually have access to the medications in this setting. If a prescriber or patient requests non-child-resistant containers, they can be provided by the pharmacist. However, a signed release form must be kept on file if a patient's medications are dispensed without child-resistant packaging. Medications that do not need to be dispensed in a child-resistant container include:

- sublingual nitroglycerin tablets
- birth control pills
- certain corticosteroid tablets
- bulky medications, such as some of the Potassium effervescent tablets

It is important to note that any prescription order that leaves the pharmacy must have a safety cap.

Occupational Safety and Health Act

Enacted in 1970, the Occupational Safety and Health Act (OSHA) was established to prevent workplace disease and injuries. It applies to almost every employer in the United States and requires them to ensure employee safety and health. It includes regulations for physical workplaces, machinery, and equipment. It also ensures that the workplace is free from recognized hazards. It provides pharmacy personnel with a set of guidelines while they work with items that can be hazardous to their health. Example agents would be a cytotoxic drug such as Cisplatin® (used in the treatment of cancer) or radioactive pharmaceutical agents such as Cardiolite® (used with Technetium Tc99m, a radioactive substance to take pictures of the heart).

Drug Listing Act

Enacted in 1972, the Drug Listing Act assigns a unique and permanent drug code to each medication. The code is known as the National Drug Code (NDC), which identifies the manufacturer, medication, and size or type of the packaging. Each medication is

assigned a code that is 11 digits long. The first 5 digits indicate manufacturer, the next 4 digits indicate the product, and the last 2 digits indicate package size. Using the NDC for verification is imperative to ensure that a medication is correct when it is dispensed. Also, when processing medications through insurance, what is being billed must match what is being filled. If the NDC of the submission does not match the dispensed product, it could be considered fraud.

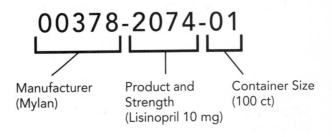

00378-2074-01

Manufacturer (Mylan)

Product and Strength (Lisinopril 10 mg)

Container Size (100 ct)

Federal Hazardous Substance Act

Enacted in 1960, the Federal Hazardous Substance Act (FHSA) involves different aspects, including the use and disposal of hazardous material in the pharmacy setting. This is mainly a concern in the hospital setting—or, more specifically, the IV room where intravenous solutions are being prepared. Any drug involving human blood or the treatment of cancer, such as anti-neoplastic drugs, must be discarded in a well-recognized puncture container marked as "Hazardous Substances." This would include anything used in the preparation of these IVs, such as personal protective equipment (PPE), or masks, gowns, gloves, etc. This act also applies to sharp equipment such as needles, which are to be disposed of in what is known as a "sharps" container.

Orphan Drug Act

Enacted in 1983, the Orphan Drug Act offers financial incentives to organizations that develop and market medications that were not previously available in the United States. Medications that treat a small part of the population are often not cost-effective to develop and market. Therefore, this act allows the treatments, called **orphan drugs**, to be developed. The act offers tax breaks and a seven-year monopoly on the drug's patent. After this act, medications like Syprine®, a chelating agent, was developed to treat the rare Wilson's Disease—which involves the body's inability to remove copper. Another example is Pamisyl®, which is used to treat ulcerative colitis.

Omnibus Budget Reconciliation Act

Enacted in 1990, the Omnibus Budget Reconciliation Act (OBRA) contains important amendments that affect both Medicare and Medicaid. This act requires pharmacies that fill prescription orders for Medicaid patients to obtain, record, and maintain basic patient information. This is an important act for pharmacy technicians, as they play an integral role in maintaining patient profiles. It also says that each state must require its pharmacists to offer counseling to patients, as well as perform what are called drug utilization reviews (DUR), which are reviews of a patient profile to ensure that medications dispensed to a patient in the past were correct. The pharmacist is also required to fix any errors found in the review.

Prescription Processing

Record Rx	
Label	
Record	
PA Request	
Refill Rx	
Refill by Rx #	
History	
Last Refill	
PA, DUR, etc.	
3rd Party	
Last Claim	
Status	
Nursing	
Pricing	
Counselling	

Rx No — 387075
Dispense Date — 02/19/10
RPh Initials — SW
Prescription Date — 02/19/10
Origin — Written

Customer | Family | Balances
Smith, Jane
456 Main Street
Anytown — AP 11111
Phone — (800) 555-555
Birthday
Insurance
Card Holder ID
Other Plan — O Insurance O Cash

Doctor
Jones, Joe
Off Phone
Fax
License
DEA #
UPIN

Prescribed
Atenolol 25 mg tablet
Avilable Drug Choices

Atenolol 25 mg tablet
Tenormin 25 mg tablet

Dispensed | History
Atenolol 25 mg tablet
Manufacture
NDC #
Package Size — 100.00
Price | Reset | GEN
AWP Cost — 21.08
Acq. Cost — 26.09
Cust. Price — 0.00
Price
Copay
Dose
Serial #

Refills Ordered
Refill #
Prescribed — 30.00
Dispensed — 30.00
Remaining — 0.00
DAW

Sig — T1T D

Sig. in English
Take 1 tablet daily

Sig. in Alternate Language

Prescribed Days Supply — 30
Dispensed Days Supply — 30
Diag Code
Rx Notes | Scan Prescription

Anabolic Steroids Control Act

Enacted in 1990, the Anabolic Steroids Control Act allows the CSA to regulate anabolic steroids. These substances promote human muscle growth and are often used illegally by athletes. These medications can have serious health consequences when abused. Under the act, anabolic steroids became a schedule III controlled substance. It also raises penalties for illegal distribution of these agents. As a technician, it is important to understand the proper indication for anabolic steroid use and report any suspected misuse to the pharmacist for proper verification.

Health Insurance Portability and Accountability Act

Enacted in 1996, the Health Insurance Portability and Accountability Act (HIPAA) was implemented to improve continuity and portability of health insurance for patients. It also sought to improve the effectiveness of Medicare and Medicaid by implementing systems to share and store private health information. The regulations are divided into three parts: privacy regulations, security regulations, and transaction standards. The privacy regulations establish patient's rights with regard to their own information. These rights include access to records, accounting of disclosures, and communication of health information. The security regulations were established to ensure the confidentiality of the **protected health information** (PHI). The transaction standards establish a common set of rules for transmitting claims. At the pharmacy level, staff must record the facility's acknowledgment of the HIPAA standards for each patient. This is maintained either in a records book or electronically through the credit card key pad found at each register. The patient will sign off that they have received the HIPAA acknowledgment and that they have no questions regarding it.

FDA Modernization Act

Enacted in 1997, the FDA Modernization Act was designed to reform the regulation of cosmetics, food, and medical products. Its main focus is safe pharmacy compounding and the regulation of medical devices. It increases the access that patients have to experimental medications and medical devices. It also mandates risk assessment reviews of products that contain mercury in the United States. The law also requires the labels of every legend medication to bear the words "Rx Only." Overall, this act improved the FDA's regulation of medications, with a focus on speeding up the approval process.

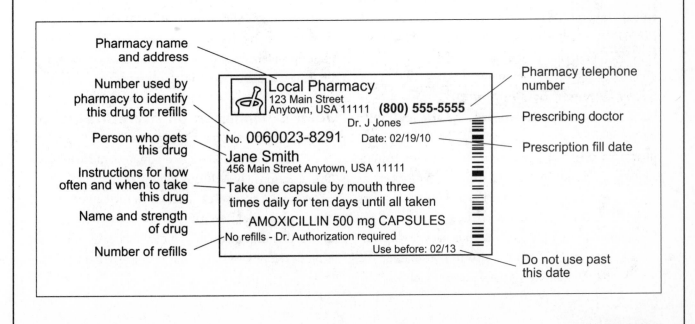

Combat Methamphetamine Epidemic Act

Enacted in 2005, the Combat Methamphetamine Epidemic Act was intended to stop the use of the illegal drug methamphetamine. This act regulates drug trafficking that is used to finance terrorism. Under this provision, any person found in violation of this act will have their property seized. Any medications named in the act, such as ephedrine and pseudoephedrine, must be kept locked up behind the pharmacy counter. The law also limits the amount of pure ephedrine or pseudoephedrine to 3.6 grams purchased per person at one time and 7.5 grams per month. Anyone who purchases a product containing ephedrine or pseudoephedrine must also furnish identification, which is registered at the pharmacy. pharmacy technicians are responsible for assisting in the maintenance of this documentation, which is entered into a national database.

Regulatory Bodies

The following are regulatory bodies that assist in the administration and enforcement of the laws related to the practice of pharmacy. These bodies function to protect the general public, patients of the pharmacy, and the pharmacy provider itself. They also help to enforce the established guidelines necessary to manufacture and distribute medications safely.

State Boards of Pharmacy

Each state has its own **state board of pharmacy** (BOP). These boards are designed to establish state-specific pharmacy laws and regulations. They are also responsible for the administration of licensure and/or certification for pharmacy personnel, which in some states includes pharmacy technicians. The state also administers board exams to license its pharmacy professionals. In addition, the board is also responsible for the oversight and discipline of these professionals.

Drug Enforcement Agency

The Drug Enforcement Agency is a federal regulatory body that is responsible for enforcing controlled substance legislation. It works to bring offenders to justice while promoting the reduction of illicit substances. The DEA works with state, local, and international agencies to execute its mission. Their focus is on major violators on the Controlled Substances Act who use violence as a part of their illegal transactions. The DEA uses assets seized from violators to help combat other targets. Since the pharmacy dispenses controlled substances, it is regulated by many laws enforced by the DEA. A pharmacy technician must understand the role of the DEA in the regulation of controlled substances so that he or she can act within those laws as well as comply with any investigation that the DEA may conduct.

Food and Drug Administration

The FDA was established to enforce the safety and effectiveness of foods, medications, biological products, cosmetics, and radioactive substances. It disseminates information about the products it regulates, with an emphasis on better, safer, and more cost-effective products. The FDA utilizes a system called **MedWatch** to receive information about adverse events or product problems. This system can be used by practitioners and patients alike. Although there are no direct penalties for not reporting information about problems to MedWatch, it is a violation of the pharmacy technician code of ethics.

Joint Commission on Accreditation of Healthcare Organizations

The Joint Commission on Accreditation of Healthcare Organizations (JCAHO) is a body that accredits and certifies healthcare organizations in the United States. This independent, not-for-profit agency works to improve safety and quality of healthcare. Its emphasis is on developing systems that increase patient safety.

National Association of the Boards of Pharmacy

The **National Association of the Boards of Pharmacy** assists the boards of pharmacy in each state to protect public health by developing uniform standards. It implements standards that reduce the likelihood of errors and public harm due to the complexities of medications.

State Laws

In many cases, pharmacy laws vary from state to state. States are responsible for establishing the minimum standards and qualifications for pharmacists and technicians in their specific jurisdictions. It is important to have an understanding of the differences between federal laws and those of the state that one is practicing in. Each state will determine how a prescription is processed and define the scope of practice for personnel and the handling of certain medications.

Although some state and federal laws may differ, in all cases the most stringent law is the one that should be followed.

Processing a Prescription

When processing a prescription, it is important to follow all steps carefully, as this is the first place where a mistake or oversight can occur. The same steps, in the same order, should be performed each time a prescription is submitted by a patient.

- Check the prescription to ensure it is valid. This includes having a patient name, date, medication name, and quantity.
- Verify the name. Ensure that the name on the prescription resembles the name the patient gives you. Some pharmacies require that the patient show a legal picture ID to authenticate the name on the prescription.

- Record the date of birth. This is for insurance processing purposes, as well as to differentiate between patients with the same name.
- Record the address. This is required to fill all controlled schedule II through V drugs, according to the Controlled Substance Act, but also helps to keep your patient profile up-to-date in the event the pharmacy needs to contact the patient.
- Record the phone number. This allows the pharmacy to contact the patient directly to provide customer service.
- Verify any patient allergies. This allows the pharmacy to ensure that the medication about to be dispensed will not harm the patient. It is also used to monitor future prescriptions to which a patient may be allergic.
- Record the insurance information. This is used for billing purposes so that a patient does not have to pay full retail price for a medication.

Entering Prescriptions

Entering prescription information is another area where an error can occur. These are usually billing or patient profile errors, but they may still be dangerous or costly. The following methods help to reduce the chance of error when entering and processing a prescription.

- When pulling up a patient profile to begin entering a prescription, make sure the entire last name is spelled out and the first letter of the first name is entered. When this is done, it will pull up a list of patients in the computer with that last name and the same first letter of the first name. You can choose the correct patient by verifying their date of birth.
- Verify insurance information. This is done when the patient presents a new insurance card.
- Search for the physician the same way a patient is found. If the wrong doctor's name is put on the prescription, there is a potential for an insurance audit or pharmacist oversight.

- Enter the name of the medication to be dispensed. There are two ways this can be done: by NDC number or by drug name. NDC is a standardized method used by all manufacturers to identify each individual drug by a sequence of numbers. All NDCs consist of 11 digits which appear like this: 12345-6789-10. The first five indicate the manufacturer, the next four indicate the drug and strength, and the last two indicate package size.

- Enter the quantity to be dispensed. This may change because of insurance purposes. Most insurance companies only cover 30 days' worth of medication at a retail pharmacy.

- Enter codes for directions in the computer. This is where another vital mistake can occur. If the pharmacy technician interprets the prescription incorrectly, it will be typed and appear on the label as such. If the pharmacist misses this mistake and dispenses it to a patient, then the patient may take an incorrect dosage and could possibly be harmed.

- Enter day supply. This is the quantity of pills, divided by how many times a day the medication is used. For example, 90 tabs/TID = 30 days. If there is an error on the part of the processing, it can lead to an insurance audit.

- Enter the number of refills. The pharmacy technician must include the exact number of refills on the prescription according to law. Note:
  - For controlled drugs, CII cannot have refills.
  - CIII to CV may have up to five refills maximum, and the prescription is good for up to six months from the date written.
  - For noncontrolled drugs, the maximum number of refills is 11, and the prescription is good for one year from the date written.

- Enter the expiration date. This must come directly from the stock bottle. If the wrong expiration date is entered, the patient could potentially take expired medication.

- Process through the patient's insurance. This is the last step and the step where the pharmacy receives authorization to dispense a drug.

Counting, Measuring, Pouring, and Labeling

Counting, measuring, pouring, and labeling may seem like simple tasks, but they have great importance within the pharmacy. This must also be done in specific steps in order to prevent errors or to allow pharmacy staff to catch any errors that have been made while processing.

- Verify that the name on the label matches the prescription. This is the first place many mistakes occur. If the names do not match, then the label is wrong and must be fixed before the pharmacy technician can continue.

- Verify that the drug on the label matches the prescription. This is another common mistake that must be caught. Both the drug and the medication strength on the label must match the prescription.

- Count the quantity of pills from the stock bottle, as indicated on the label. Make sure the NDCs match on both the bottle and the label. If they do not, the label must be changed. The pharmacy technician must always bill exactly what is being filled. This ensures that the stock indicated in the computer matches what is contained on the shelves.

- Place the medication in a vial, then attach the label. This is a very important step because if the wrong label is attached to the wrong vial, it can cause the patient to take a medication the wrong way; and since the prescription would match a label on a bottle, it could cause the pharmacist to possibly overlook that the medication didn't match.

Prescription Drug Orders

Each state has laws that regulate the prescribers of medications. Each practitioner must be state licensed and if prescribing narcotics, registered with the DEA as well. In some states, nurse practitioners, physician assistants, and even pharmacists can prescribe medications. If a prescription is for a controlled substance, it must include all the information that a regular prescription includes, as well as an address for the patient and a DEA number given to the physician to write for controlled schedule drugs. The prescription must also be hand-signed, not stamped.

Labeling

Although each practice setting has its own labeling requirements, federal standard requirements are as follows. A single-unit package of an individual dose or unit dose products must include:

- medication name (trade or generic)
- route of administration, if it is not oral
- strength and volume of medication
- medication's lot number and expiration date
- repackager's name or license number
- special storage information

Multiple-use medication packages must include:

- identifying information about the dispensing pharmacy
- patient's name
- dispensing date
- medication name and strength

Ambulatory, or outpatient, packages must include:

- name and address of dispensing pharmacy
- patient's name
- prescriber's information
- directions for use
- dispensing date
- federal or state cautions
- prescription number
- name or initials of dispensing pharmacist
- name and strength of the medication
- manufacturer's name
- expiration date

Patient Records and Drug Review

The maintenance of a patient's records helps monitor drug therapies effectively. It is also documentation of what has and has not been done with regard to the patient. It should contain the patient's full name, address and telephone number(s), age or birth date, and gender. Every pharmacy should also ensure that they have their patient's entire medication history. This will help to identify duplicate or contraindicated therapies. It is the pharmacist's responsibility to review all patient profiles for misuse or abuse by doing a drug utilization review under OBRA. Although the pharmacy technician is not directly responsible for this review, he or she is expected to bring any suspected misuse or abuse to the pharmacist's attention.

Patient Counseling

Patient counseling can only be performed by a licensed pharmacist. Under OBRA, most states have established a mandatory counseling law. Counseling is an effective tool in preventing errors, as it gives the patient and provider an opportunity to discuss the treatment and the possibility of adverse reactions. It also gives the pharmacist the chance to answer any questions a patient may have regarding the medication. It is important to understand that a pharmacy technician may do almost all duties required in the pharmacy setting except for those that require an educated judgment decision. In the case of the counseling of patients, pharmacy technicians should not be doing this.

Sale of Hypodermic Needles and Syringes

The sale of hypodermic needles or syringes must be controlled by the pharmacist to prevent their illegal use. Each state regulates the over-the-counter sale of these products to persons 18 years and older, with some requiring a written prescription from the physician. In addition, pharmacies are not to advertise the fact that they sell needles and syringes; and the purchase may be limited to ten per day, depending upon state law.

Practice Questions

1. Which of the following is not a category in the legal system?
   a. criminal law
   b. civil law
   c. contract law
   d. malicious law

2. The core of our laws comes from the U.S. Constitution. Which of the following laws is derived from the judicial branch of the government, or court system?
   a. constitutional law
   b. legislative law
   c. administrative law
   d. common law

3. Of the following DEA numbers, which one is correct if the physician's name is Dr. Tim Longley?
   a. AL4317651
   b. AT4317651
   c. AL4317653
   d. AT4317653

4. The FDA utilizes a system called _____ to receive information about adverse events or product problems.
   a. Phase I Marketing
   b. Phase II Marketing
   c. Phase III Marketing
   d. MedWatch

5. Which of the following is a CII controlled substance?
   a. Vicodin®
   b. Oxybutnin®
   c. Percocet®
   d. Darvocet-N®

6. Which of the following acts is a crime that may result in criminal prosecution?
   a. falsifying information when applying for a license
   b. failure to provide reasonable care
   c. practicing without a license
   d. all of the above

7. Of the following regulatory agencies, which one deals with regulation of healthcare organizations, such as a pharmacy in a hospital setting?
   a. FDA
   b. JCAHO
   c. DEA
   d. HIPPA

8. Laws which are prescribed by legislative acts are known as
   a. administrative law.
   b. case law.
   c. statutory law.
   d. common law.

9. Of the following schedules of drugs, which one is considered to have no medicinal value?
   a. schedule I
   b. schedule II
   c. schedule III
   d. schedule V

10. The _____ requires the proper labeling or branding of products and also requires that the contents of a container cannot be changed from what they are labeled to be.
    a. PPPA
    b. FD&C Act
    c. Hazardous Substance Labeling Act
    d. Orphan Drug Act

11. Which of the following is a main consideration of the pharmacy technician code of ethics?
    a. preventing the patient from dying
    b. prevention of communicable diseases
    c. health and safety of the patient
    d. patients' ability to afford medications

12. The PPPA requires
    a. the use of safety caps for all new prescription orders in a retail pharmacy.
    b. patient counseling for all new prescription orders received in a retail pharmacy.
    c. that all drug manufacturer containers be labeled correctly as to what is inside the container.
    d. that drugs within a drug manufacturer's container not be adulterated.

13. For the following NDC number, what would the first set of numbers be indicative of?

    NDC: 50111-0648-03

    a. the product
    b. the manufacturer
    c. the package size
    d. the generic name

14. Lack of attention to detail or any distractions can contribute to which of the following situations?
    a. professional ethics violations
    b. conflicts of interest
    c. social problems
    d. errors and mistakes

15. Enacted in 2005, the Combat Methamphetamine Epidemic Act was intended to stop the use of the illegal drug methamphetamine by limiting the sales of what drug?
    a. phenylpropanolamine
    b. pseudoephedrine
    c. caffeine
    d. ranitidine

16. At the pharmacy level, they must record the acknowledgment of the facility's _____ standards for each new patient.
    a. OBRA
    b. SARS
    c. HIPPA
    d. PPPA

17. According to CSA, schedule II drugs are not allowed any refills. What is the maximum number of refills a CII through CV can have, and how long is the prescription valid after the date of issue?
    a. 5 refills and six months
    b. 11 refills and one year
    c. 6 refills and one year
    d. 11 refills and six months

18. Which of the following statements is true?
    a. A pharmacy technician can be held accountable and liable in a court of law for a medication error.
    b. In some states, pharmacy technicians are allowed to counsel patients.
    c. A pharmacy technician cannot be held accountable and liable in a court of law for a medication error.
    d. If the pharmacist feels the technician is qualified, the technician need not have filled prescriptions checked by the pharmacist.

19. Any questions or situations involving controlled drugs should be directed to which regulatory agency?
    a. FDA
    b. BOP
    c. DEA
    d. HIPPA

20. Which state regulatory agency is responsible for the administration of licensure and/or certification of pharmacy personnel?
   a. FDA
   b. BOP
   c. DEA
   d. HIPPA

21. Of the following, which one accredits and certifies healthcare organizations in the United States?
   a. OSHA
   b. JCAHO
   c. NABP
   d. BOP

22. Comprehensive Drug Abuse Prevention and Control Act is also known as the
   a. Poison Prevention Packaging Act.
   b. Federal Drug and Cosmetic Act.
   c. Controlled Substance Act.
   d. Omnibus Budget Reconciliation Act.

23. Which of the following is a CIV controlled substance?
   a. Vicodin®
   b. Oxybutnin®
   c. Percocet®
   d. Zolpidem®

24. The Orphan Drug Act deals with drugs that are
   a. outdated.
   b. used to treat rare disease states.
   c. used to treat syndromes.
   d. used to treat type II diabetes mellitus.

25. For the following prescription medication, what is the maximum number of refills allowed?

Lisinopril 10 mg #120
sig: i po tid

   a. 3
   b. 5
   c. 11
   d. 12

Answers and Explanations

1. d. Criminal law is enforced by a state representative against persons or companies. In civil law, a plaintiff will bring a suit against an alleged defendant. Contract law is an agreement between two or more parties and is typically enforced in civil court.

2. d. Constitutional law is drawn from the U.S. Constitution and the Bill of Rights. Legislative law is drawn from the legislative branch of the government. Administrative law is derived from the executive branch of the government (the president or state governor and their cabinets).

3. a. The DEA number for physicians consists of two letters, the first letter of which is either an A or B. The second letter is the first letter of the physician's last name. These letters are followed by seven numbers, the sequence of which can easily be solved: $4 + 1 + 6 = 11$; $3 + 7 + 5 = 15$; $(15)(2) = 30$; $11 + 30 = 31$.

4. d. MedWatch is done after a drug is marketed to the public as a way to obtain information from patients who may have concerns about the new medication they are taking. There is no such thing as a Phase I, II, or III Marketing.

5. c. Percocet® Vicodin® is a schedule III drug; Oxybutnin® is a noncontrolled drug; Darvocet-N® is a schedule III drug.

6. d. All of these acts are punishable crimes.

7. b. FDA deals with drug regulations, DEA deals with controlled drugs, and HIPPA deals with patient confidentiality. JCAHO regulates pharmacies in the hospital setting.

8. c. Statutory law is prescribed by legislative enactments. Administrative law is enacted by the president, while case law and common law are based on court decisions.

9. a. Schedule I drugs are considered to have no medicinal value and are not dispensed in the pharmacy setting.

10. b. PPPA deals with safety caps for prescription drugs. Hazardous Substance Labeling Act deals with the use of a hazardous container for hazardous materials. Orphan Drug Act deals with drugs that are used for rare disease states. The FD&C Act is the correct answer.

11. c. The goal of the code is to ensure patient health and safety. Although the other items are important considerations, they are not directly covered in the code.

12. a. PPPA stands for the Poison Prevention Packaging Act, so the most appropriate answer is the use of safety caps.

13. b. The NDC number consists of three sets of digits. The first set of digits is indicative of the manufacturer. The second set of digits would be what the drug product is, and the third set would be indicative of the package size.

14. d. Lack of attention will cause mistakes or errors.

15. b. Pseudoephedrine is the generic name for Sudafed®. Phenylpropanolamine was removed from the market due to addiction concerns. Caffeine is also of concern but will never be removed from the market. Ranitidine is the generic name for Zantac®, which is used for GERD.

16. c. HIPPA deals with patient confidentiality. All new customers in a pharmacy setting are given a protected health information (PHI) form that details the pharmacy's stance on this issue.

17. a. A schedule III to schedule V drug is allowed to have 5 refills, with the prescription being valid for six months from the date of issue. Noncontrolled legend (prescription) drugs are allowed a maximum of 11 refills, with the prescription being valid for one year from date of issue. Schedule II drugs cannot be refilled.

18. a. With the new roles established for pharmacy technicians, which includes the filling of prescription and medication orders, a pharmacy technician *can* be held liable in a court of law.

19. c. FDA regulates the marketing of drugs, BOP regulates pharmacies within their state, HIPPA deals with patient confidentiality. The DEA regulates controlled substances.

20. b. BOP regulates administration of licensure and/or certification of pharmacy personnel. The FDA deals with getting drugs to the market that are safe and effective. The DEA regulated schedule drugs that are part of the Controlled Substance Act. HIPPA is a federal law that mandates patient confidentiality.

21. b. The Joint Commission accredits and certifies healthcare organizations in the United States. OSHA deals with safety requirements in all work settings, NABP is the National Association Board of Pharmacies which regulates individual state boards of pharmacies, and BOP is an individual state board of pharmacy that regulates pharmacies within their state and administration of licensure and/or certification of pharmacy personnel.

22. c. The Controlled Substance Act. The PPPA deals with the mandated issuance of safety caps in the pharmacy setting. The FD&C Act deals with labeling and adulteration of a drug, and OBRA deals with the need to do DURs and the counseling of Medicaid patients.

23. d. Zolpidem or Ambien®. Sleep aids are generally schedule IV drugs, as are anti-anxiety aids that belong to the drug classification called benzodiazepines.

24. b. The Orphan Drug Act offers financial incentives to develop medications for rare disease states. The other options have nothing to do with the Orphan Drug Act.

25. c. Lisinipril is a noncontrolled drug used for hypertension or high blood pressure. The maximum number of refills is 11 for noncontrolled drugs. For controlled schedule II drugs, there are no refills allowed, and for controlled schedule III through V drugs, the maximum number of refills is 5.

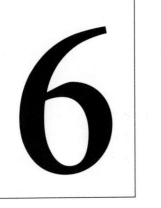

6 ▶ Dosage Forms and Routes of Administration

CHAPTER OVERVIEW

In the pharmacy setting, you will see different types of formulations, or dosage forms, of manufactured drugs which are dependent on the route of administration, absorption, and practicality. You will see solid dosage forms (which would include tablets, capsules, lozenges, powders, and granules), as well as liquid dosage formulations (which would include solutions, elixirs, and suspensions). In this chapter, we will look at all of the above, as well as parenteral routes of administration (those formulations which bypass the digestive system). Finally, we will identify special considerations for each route of administration as well as the advantages and disadvantages of specific formulations.

KEY TERMS

additive	diluent	extended-release
aerosol	dosage form	film-coated
ampoule (also ampule)	douche	hydro-alcoholic
buccal	effervescent	gargle
capsule	elixir	hydrophilic
chewable	enema	inhalation
cream	enteric-coated	inhaler
delayed-release	excipient	injection

KEY TERMS (continued)

intraocular	parenteral	suspension
irrigation	pellet	syrup
liquid	powder	tablet
lotion	preservative	tincture
lozenge	propellant	topical
mucilage	rectal	transdermal
nasal	solution	troches
ointment	spray	vaginal
ophthalmic	subcutaneous	vial
oral	sublingual	wash
otic	suppository	

Medication Dosage Forms

Drugs are seldom administered in pure form. They are formulated into a variety of dosage forms to facilitate administration, effectiveness, and safety. A **dosage form** is a system or device for delivering the drug to the body. In a dosage form, the active ingredient, referred to as the drug or medication, is combined with inert (or inactive) materials that facilitate administration of the drug.

Dosage form means different things to different people. A patient thinks of a dosage form as the gross, final product represented by a **tablet**, **capsule**, or **liquid** formulation. Members of the healthcare team think of a dosage form as the drug-delivery system. Changes in any part of the drug-delivery system, including changes in inactive or inert ingredients, may alter the delivery rate and the total amount of the drug delivered to the site of action in the patient's body.

The formulation of contents inside various dosage forms may include:

- **additives:** additional formulation aids that may be necessary for a successful preparation of the dosage form
- **diluents:** additives used to increase the bulk weight or volume of a dosage form so that the dose of the active drug is more easily handled by the patient
- **excipients:** inactive substances used as a carrier for the active ingredients of a medication
- **preservatives:** substances that retard, minimize, or prevent the growth of bacteria or other microorganisms in the dosage form

Most drugs today are synthesized and, in pure form, are solid powders or crystals. Some drugs, however, may exist only in liquid or gas state. A solid drug can be formulated into a solid or liquid final product, but a liquid drug can only be made into a liquid dosage form—unless the dose of the drug is very small. If the dose of the drug is extremely small (for example, a few drops), sometimes it can be absorbed into a dry powder, with the dosage formulated as a solid. A drug in a gas state can be formulated only into a gaseous dosage form.

Because of the varied physical character of drugs, their mode of action, and the route of administration used for delivery, dosage forms may be classified in several different ways. For our purposes, the major classes of drug dosage forms may be broadly categorized into four main classes: solid, liquid, semisolid, and miscellaneous dosage forms.

Solid Dosage Forms

Solid dosage forms include tablets, **suppositories**, and various types of **lozenges**. **Powders** and granules are also solid dosage forms, but they comprise a very small part of solid dosage forms dispensed today. A solid dosage form (such as tablets and capsules) offers several advantages and has gained popularity because it has:

- increased stability, yielding longer shelf life
- ease of packaging, storage, dispensing, and transporting
- accurate dosing due to its pre-divided forms
- controlled-release characteristics
- convenience for self-administration
- little or no taste or smell, in most cases

However, solid dosage forms are not without disadvantages. They may be difficult to swallow, cannot be used in unconscious patients, have a slow onset of action, and may be degraded by acid in the stomach.

Capsules

Capsules are a solid dosage form where the drug (with or without inert ingredients) is enclosed within a gelatin shell. The gelatin dissolves in the stomach after approximately 10–30 minutes, releasing the drug. Capsule dosage forms are available as hard or soft gelatin capsules. There are a wide variety of distinguishable capsule shapes and colors on the market. In fact, the dosage form is popular because of this trait.

A hard gelatin capsule consists of a two-piece, unsealed, oblong casing filled with powdered ingredients. The contents of a hard gelatin capsule may range from 50 mg to 1 g of powder per capsule. Hard gelatin capsules should be stored in airtight containers under controlled relative humidity (less than 10%), or they may stick together. They are usually swallowed whole but may be opened and sprinkled on food or inhaled using a special administration device. *Examples: Amoxil® (swallowed), Theo-Dur® (sprinkled on food), Ventolin Rotacaps® (inhaled).*

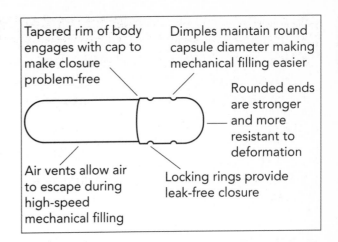

Tapered rim of body engages with cap to make closure problem-free

Dimples maintain round capsule diameter making mechanical filling easier

Rounded ends are stronger and more resistant to deformation

Air vents allow air to escape during high-speed mechanical filling

Locking rings provide leak-free closure

Soft gelatin capsules contain additives that give the gelatin a soft, squeezable, elastic consistency. The two halves of the capsule are sealed shut. The shape of the capsule may be round, elliptical, or oblong, and it is filled with liquid, pastes, or powders. If filled with liquid, it should be nonaqueous, because the presence of water will soften or dissolve the gelatin shell. The contents of a soft gelatin capsule range from 1 mL to almost 3 mL. *Examples: Colace®, vitamin A, and Marinol®.*

Sizes of capsules range from,000 (largest) to 5 (smallest). Capsule size,000 is generally too large to be swallowed by most patients, but it can be used when the contents of the capsule are emptied and mixed with a liquid or food. The volume of powder that can be placed in a given capsule varies and depends on two factors: the density of the powder being placed in the empty capsule and the degree to which the powder can be compacted.

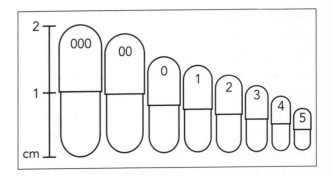

There is a wide variety of advantages to capsule dosage forms, because:

- it is easy to carry the day's supply
- they are easy to swallow
- it is easy to identify a product because of the wide range of colors
- it is easy to mask undesirable taste and/or odor, because the shell is tasteless
- they are flexible for providing combination drugs
- they are easy to produce economically in large quantities

Tablets

Tablets are drug solids formed in molds or by die punch compression. They may also include inert (inactive) ingredients such as binders, diluents, lubricants, colors, disintegrators, sweeteners, and flavors. These inert ingredients are termed *excipients* and do not possess any therapeutic activity. Tablets may also have a coating applied to the outside to mask unpleasant flavor and/or odor, or to protect the drug from stomach contents. They are the most popular of all medicinal preparations intended for oral use. Tablets offer the advantages of accurate dosage, a compact dosage form, portability, the convenience of self-administration, and a bland taste. Examples include HydroDIURIL® and Synthroid®.

Although frequently discoid (flat and round) in form, tablets are available in various shapes and sizes, including round, triangular, oblong, cylindrical, bullet, square, diamond, almond, oval, and even capsule-shaped. Color is generally included in the formulation for identification or visual appeal. Some tablets are scored, so that they may be easily broken in halves or quarters. However, some tablets designed for extended- or sustained-release should never be broken or crushed. These drugs would generally have an abbreviation following the drug name to indicate that the formulation is meant for extended or sustained release, such as XL, XR, LA, SR, etc. Example drugs: Entex LA, Effexor XR, Cardizem SR.

Most tablet dosage forms are embossed with the name of the manufacturer or a tablet code number for identification.

In addition to the traditional tablets, there are a variety of specialized tablet formulations:

- **Chewable** tablets are designed to be chewed before swallowing. This formulation is usually pleasantly flavored and useful for children or adult patients who cannot swallow easily. They may be dissolved in the mouth or swallowed intact. *Examples: baby aspirin, Tums®, Gaviscon®.*
- **Enteric-coated** (EC) tablets are coated with a substance to prevent dissolution in the acid environment of the stomach. They are meant to dissolve in the intestine, in order to protect the drug against acid in the stomach or to protect the stomach lining against the drug. EC dosage forms may never be chewed, broken, or crushed prior to ingestion or taken with antacids. *Examples: ECASA, Dulcolax®.*
- **Sublingual** tablets are designed to dissolve quickly under the tongue so that the active ingredient is rapidly absorbed. Since absorption does not rely on the gastrointestinal tract, the active ingredient avoids early metabolism in the liver. *Example: nitroglycerin, Isordil®.*
- **Buccal** tablets are designed to be placed between the cheek and gum, where the drug dissolves slowly over a period. *Example: Fentanyl Oralet®.*
- **Film-coated** tablets are usually coated with a thin layer of water-soluble material that dissolves rapidly in the stomach. The purpose of the coating is to cover an unpleasant taste or smell, or to protect sensitive drugs from deterioration due to the effects of air and light. *Example: erythromycin.*
- **Effervescent** tablets contain sodium bicarbonate and citric and/or tartaric acid so that when the drug is placed in liquid, an acid-base reaction causes carbon dioxide gas bubbles and releases the active drug. The tablet quickly disintegrates and dissolves before administration. The dosage form affords rapid drug absorption because the drug is dissolved before it reaches the stomach. *Example: Alka-Seltzer®.*

- **Pellets** are small, cylinder-shaped tablets meant for implantation beneath the skin. They provide prolonged, continuous drug absorption of potent hormones. *Examples: testosterone, estradiol.*
- **Vaginal** tablets are designed to be inserted into the vagina, where they dissolve, and the active drug is absorbed through the vaginal lining. The product may come with an applicator to facilitate insertion. *Example: Gyne-Lotrimin®.*

Lozenges

Lozenges are hard, oval, or discoid solid dosage forms with a drug contained in a flavored sugar base. They dissolve slowly to keep the drug in prolonged contact with the mouth or throat. Typically, they contain antiseptic, anesthetic, antibiotic, astringent, analgesic, or antitussive (cough suppressant) drugs. They are also called troches or pastilles. *Examples: Sucrets®, Cepacol®, Mycelex®.*

Suppositories

Suppositories are designed for insertion into the rectum, vaginal cavity, or urethral tract. Suppositories designed for insertion into the vagina are sometimes referred to as inserts, particularly when the suppository is made by compression into specially shaped tablets.

The rectal suppository base is an inactive ingredient, which carries the active drug and melts or dissolves in the body cavity, releasing the medication over a prolonged period of time. The effect may be local or systemic (throughout the body). Instruct the patients to unwrap the suppository before inserting. *Examples: Bisacodyl, Compazine®, B&O Supprettes.*

Powders

Powders are finely ground mixtures of dry drugs and inactive ingredients which are sprinkled or dusted on the area to be treated (for example, Mycostatin® powder). When used internally, they are usually dissolved in water prior to ingestion (for example, potassium supplements). Some are mixed with water and used in the wet state (for example, tooth powders).

Granules

Granules are powders that are wetted, allowed to dry, and ground into course, irregular pieces. The particle size is larger than powders, and the granules are usually more stable. Water may be added to prepare a **solution** or suspension at the time of dispensing (as with oral antibiotic suspensions like Senokot®). Effervescent granules release a gas (usually carbon dioxide) when placed in water, which facilitates dissolution and helps mask the taste of salty or bitter medications.

Liquid Dosage Forms Containing Soluble Matter

Drugs in a molecular form cause biological responses; the body responds when drug molecules interact with receptors in the body. Thus, no matter whether a drug is administered in solid, liquid, or gas form, the action at the receptor level will involve an interaction with individual molecules of the drug. Therefore, for any drug to cause the desired effect, it has to be present in the form of a molecular solution at the site of action. Liquid dosage forms (solutions, emulsions, suspensions, etc.) are often the dosage form of choice because they are:

- effective more quickly than a solid dosage form because the solid dosage form has to dissolve before absorption
- easier to swallow, especially for pediatric and geriatric patients
- easier to place down a feeding tube or injection
- flexible in dosing
- used where solid dosage forms are not practical (eye, ear)
- given in larger doses than can be formulated in tablets and capsules

As with any other dosage form, liquid dosage forms have some disadvantages as well. The following disadvantages are common to almost all liquid dosage forms:

- deterioration and loss of potency, which occurs much faster than the corresponding solid dosage form
- flavoring and sweetening problems with liquid dosage forms, which make it difficult to hide bitter taste or offensive odor
- higher incidence of incompatibility
- the need for added preservatives because liquid doses provide an excellent medium for growth of microorganisms
- the need for special handling or storage, such as shaking before use or refrigeration
- the potential for dosing inaccuracy if the patient uses a household measuring device, such as a teaspoon
- inconvenient to carry (due to being bulkier than solid forms) and the need to carry a measuring device

Liquid dosage forms deliver medication in a fluid medium called the vehicle (water, alcohol, or mineral oil). The drug may be dissolved in the vehicle or suspended as very fine particles. The fluid may pour freely or be thick like syrup. The dosage form may be for oral consumption, for use in or on other parts of the body, or for **injection**.

Solutions

Solutions are homogenous (evenly distributed) mixtures of one or more dissolved medications (solute) in a liquid vehicle (solvent). The dissolved drug may be solid, liquid, or gas. Active ingredients are quickly absorbed by the stomach, skin, or other site of administration. Solutions exist for both internal and external use; they should be stored so that solutions for external use are not accidentally administered orally. Aqueous solutions contain water as the solvent and include the following types:

- **douches:** directed into a body cavity to remove debris or disinfect. *Example: Massengill®.*
- **irrigations:** used to wash eyes, the urinary bladder, or open wounds; larger volumes and larger areas than douches. *Example: Neosporin® GU.*
- **enemas:** introduced into the rectum to empty the bowel or treat disease. *Example: Fleet®.*
- **gargles:** solutions that treat diseases of the throat; not swallowed. *Example: Chloraseptic®.*
- **washes:** used to cleanse or bathe a body part, such as eyes or mouth; not swallowed. *Examples: Scope®, Listerine®.*
- **sprays:** solutions delivered as a mist against the mucous membranes of the nose and throat. *Examples: Afrin®, Neo-Synephrine®.*
- **injection:** a sterile drug solution introduced beneath the skin, into the muscle, or into the bloodstream. *Example: dextrose 5% in water (D5W).*

Viscous (thick) aqueous solutions include:

- **syrups:** concentrated mixture of sugar (or artificial sweetener) and drug; often used in pediatrics. *Examples: Robitussin®, Triaminic®.*
- **mucilages:** thick, adhesive liquids containing pulpy components of vegetable matter. *Example: Metamucil®.*

Nonaqueous Solutions

Nonaqueous solutions include **hydro-alcoholic** (with water) and alcoholic solutions. The alcohol may facilitate drug dissolution, but it may also interact with other drugs the patient is taking. Special care should be exercised when dispensing hydro-alcoholic or alcoholic solutions to pediatric, elderly, and alcohol-dependent patients. They or their caregivers should be made aware of the alcohol content.

Hydro-alcoholic solutions include **elixirs** and **tinctures**. Elixirs are sweetened with a pleasant taste, have good relative stability, and are easy to prepare.

The concentration of alcohol is usually 3–25%. *Examples: Donnatal®, digoxin, phenobarbital.*

Tinctures are prepared from vegetable, animal, or chemical materials and have higher alcohol content than elixirs. *Examples: tincture of opium, tincture of iodine, tincture of paregoric.*

Alcoholic solutions contain no water because the drug is dissolved directly in ethyl alcohol. *Example: collodion.*

Liquid Dosage Forms Containing Insoluble Matter

Some drugs do not dissolve in the solvents that are commonly used to prepare liquid dosage forms; these drugs cannot be formulated as solutions. In order to obtain some of the advantages of giving a liquid dosage form, insoluble solutes may be suspended in a suitable liquid. There are two common dosage forms that do not possess adequate solubility to be formulated as solutions: emulsions and suspensions.

Emulsions

Emulsions are mixtures of two liquids that normally do not mix (e.g., oil and water). In an emulsion, one liquid is broken into small particles and evenly scattered throughout the other. The liquid present in small particles is called the internal phase, and the other liquid is called the external, or continuous, phase. The two liquids will separate into two phases unless an emulsifying agent is used. Examples of emulsifying agents include gelatin, acacia, and synthetic compounds that reduce the tension between the immiscible liquids. An emulsifying agent is a chemical that has a water-loving head on one end of the molecule and a lipid-loving tail on the other, and therefore keeps the oil and water together.

Suspensions

Suspensions are mixtures of very fine particles of an insoluble (undissolved) solid (called the internal or dispersed phase) distributed through a gas, liquid, or solid (called the dispersion or external phase). The external phase in most pharmaceutical suspensions is water, and the suspension is called an *aqueous suspension.*

Suspensions are used for drugs that are not readily soluble (able to dissolve). Usually the particles are made very fine, because fine particles dissolve in the stomach and are absorbed by the body more quickly. Suspensions need to be shaken prior to use; always affix a "shake well" auxiliary label when dispensing. Suspensions may be for oral, topical, or injectable use.

Examples of oral suspensions include oral antibiotics such as amoxicillin, which normally contain 125–500 mg of the solid drug per 5 mL (a teaspoonful) of suspension.

Injectable suspensions allow for insoluble drugs to be administered in a suitable form for intramuscular or **subcutaneous** purposes. Injectable suspensions are used for depot therapy, where the drug is released over a long period of time. Examples of depot therapy drugs include procaine penicillin G and Neutral Protamine Hagedorn (NPH) insulin.

Well-formulated suspensions have the following characteristics:

- The suspended material should not settle rapidly and should disperse readily into a uniform (evenly distributed) mixture when the container is shaken.
- It should pour freely from the orifice of the bottle—or if it is in an injectable formulation, it should pass easily through a syringe needle.
- For external application, the product must be fluid enough to spread easily over the affected area, but not be so mobile that it runs off the surface.
- External suspensions applied externally should dry quickly after application.
- External suspensions should provide an elastic protective film that will not rub off easily.
- External suspensions should have an acceptable color and odor.

Types of **suspensions** also include **lotions**, which are intended for external use; they cool, soothe, dry, or protect skin. *Example: Calamine® lotion.*

Miscellaneous Liquid Dosage Forms

Enemas are a liquid dosage form introduced into the rectum via a bulb syringe. Their action can be local or systemic. The enema solution should be at room temperature when introduced, to prevent side effects. *Example: Fleet®.*

Douches are aqueous solutions that are directed against a body part or into a cavity of the body. Eye douches remove foreign objects or discharges from the eye. Pharyngeal and **nasal** douches cleanse or soothe the nose or throat. Vaginal douches cleanse and provide medication to the vaginal mucosa.

Extended– and Delayed–Release Dosage Forms

Extended-release dosage forms are formulated so that active ingredients are released at a constant rate for a prolonged period (usually 8–24 hours). They are commonly referred to as long-acting, timed-release, delayed-release, or prolonged-action, and are typically tablets or capsules—but may include injections, implants, **troches**, or patches. **Extended-release** forms deliver medication in a slow, controlled, and consistent manner, reducing the risk of drug side effects. They are taken less frequently during the day, with better patient compliance. They may also be less costly to the patient.

Extended-release technology includes small beads in varying sizes, with differing coating thicknesses (Contac®), a slowly eroding matrix (Slow-K), leaching from an inert matrix (Procanbid®), an osmotic pump (Procardia® XL), semi-permeable membrane in a patch (Duragesic® patch), implants, injections of suspensions, medicated contact lenses, and ocular inserts.

Delayed-release dosage forms release their drug at a later time, well after administration. Enteric-coated dosage forms are an example of delayed-release dosages.

Compared to immediate-release dosage forms, extended-release dosage forms offer many advantages, including the following:

- elimination of fluctuations (jumps) of drug level in the blood during chronic (long term) administration
- reduction in adverse side effects
- reduction in frequency of administration
- enhanced patient compliance

Common abbreviations for extended-release formulations include the following:

- CD: controlled diffusion
- CR: controlled (or continuous) release
- CRT: controlled-release tablet
- LA: long-acting
- SA: sustained-action
- SR: sustained (or slow) release
- TD: time delay
- TR: time release
- XL: extra-long
- XR: extended-release

Semisolid Dosage Forms

Semisolid dosage forms are ones that are too thick or viscous to be considered a liquid dosage form, yet not solid enough to be considered a solid dosage form. These semisolid dosage forms are intended for **topical** application. They may be applied to skin, placed on mucous membranes, or used in one of the body cavities (e.g., nasal, rectal, or vaginal cavity). The most commonly used semisolid dosage forms are **ointments**, **creams**, and pastes.

- Ointments are semisolid preparations used for external application to the skin or mucous membranes. They may be vehicles for the topical application of drugs or serve as emollients (lubricating agents) or as a skin protectant. With the exception of nitroglycerin ointment, very few ointments are designed to produce systemic (whole body) effects. Ophthalmic (eye) ointments must be sterile. All ointments should have a "for external use only" auxiliary label attached before dispensing. An example would be Cortisporin Eye ointment. *Examples: FML® Eye, Elocon®.*

- Creams are semisolid emulsions containing suspensions or solutions of drugs intended for external application. They may be water-in-oil or oil-in-water emulsions. All creams require a "for external use only" label. *Examples: Kenalog®, Valisone®.*

- Pastes are ointment-like preparations for external application that are usually stiffer, less greasy, and more hydrophilic (water based) than ointments. They are applied to oozing, weeping lesions because of their ability to absorb water. All pastes should have a "for external use only" label. *Examples: Kenalog® Dental paste, Oralone® paste.*

- Gels are a two-phase system consisting of a solid internal phase diffused throughout a viscous liquid phase. By weight, gels are mostly liquid, yet they behave like solids due to a three-dimensional cross-linked network within the liquid. It is the cross-links within the fluid that give a gel its structure (hardness) and contribute to stickiness. Gels should have "for external use only" labels attached prior to dispensing. Gels include semisolid solutions used as lubricants. *Examples: K-Y® Jelly, Xylocaine® Viscous.*

- Inhalers contain solutions or suspensions of solid or liquid particles in gas or air. The drug may also be contained in a gelatin capsule, placed into an inhaler, and punctured before use. They are intended for inhalation via the nose or mouth. Inhalers should have a "shake well before use" label attached before dispensing. *Examples: Ventolin® inhaler, Azmacort® inhaler.*

Miscellaneous Dosage Forms

Aerosols are suspensions of very fine liquid or solid drug particles in a gas propellant and packaged under pressure. An aerosol dosage form consists of three components: the product concentrate, the container, and the propellant. A valve assembly allows the propellant to push the contents of the aerosol from within the container into the atmosphere. The pressurized aerosol containers should be stored away from heat. The medication may be released as a spray, foam, or solid. This dosage form delivers the drug to internal or external sites. It has a rapid onset of action because the drug bypasses the gastrointestinal or GI tract.

Aerosols offer convenience and easy application. Using an aerosol eliminates the irritation produced in the mechanical application of the drug, especially over an abraded area. Aerosol medications can also be applied to areas that are otherwise difficult to reach. *Examples: Bactine®, ProctoFoam-HC®, Tinactin®.*

Metered-dose inhalers (MDI) are used in inhalation therapy for potent medications. An accurate, fixed amount of drug is delivered with a single depression of the actuator. *Examples: Advair®, Aerobid®, and Ventolin®.*

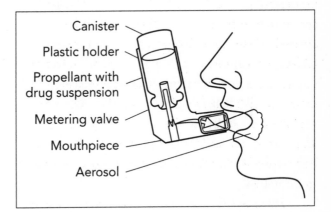

Canister
Plastic holder
Propellant with drug suspension
Metering valve
Mouthpiece
Aerosol

Metered Dose Inhaler

Injectable Dosage Forms

Injectable dosage forms are marketed in **vials**, **ampoules** (also known as **ampules**), pre-filled syringes, and pre-filled infusion bags.

- Additive vials usually come in sizes ranging from 2 ml to 50 ml. A vial will either be single dose, which is meant for the withdrawal of just one dose before the vial is discarded, or multi-dose, which is meant to be pierced by a needle for multiple doses. A vial will have the medication name on it, as well as necessary information like concentration, stability, usage directions, expiration date, and lot number, etc.

Some vials will come in a powder formulation and will need to have diluents (solution) added before administration. The rationale for powder vials is that the stability of the drug is short; once diluents are added, it will have a very short expiration date. The addition of a diluent to a powder vial is called reconstitution. The vial will give information as to which diluents should be added and how much is needed to attain a specific concentration. Always remember to clean the port using isopropyl alcohol 70% pads before piercing the rubber (diaphragm) top of the vial.

- Ampules are self-enclosed glass containers that contain sterile drugs for injection into an IV bag. Ampules can easily be opened at the neck (top), but removal of their contents must be done by a filter needle or straw. Once medication is removed, then the filter needle or straw must be replaced with a regular needle before injecting into an IV bag. The rationale for using the filter needle or straw is that once an ampule is broken, it will leave microscopic glass shards. The filter needle or straw will take out anything greater than five microns.
- Pre-filled syringes or pre-filled infusion bags will have the medication ready to be administered, as it will be in the correct solution.

Routes of Administration

A particular dosage form often implies a specific route (and vice versa). Many drugs are available in a variety of dosage forms and may be delivered via a number of routes. *Examples: steroids and antibiotics.*

Sometimes combinations of routes are used simultaneously. The oral route is most common but not always the most convenient; drugs may be administered into any orifice, through the skin, or via an artificially made opening.

Oral

Drugs administered orally are administered through the mouth and swallowed. The **oral** route is abbreviated *PO* (*per os*). *Examples: tablets, capsules, solutions, suspensions, emulsions, powders.*

Advantages of the oral route are that it is safe and convenient, the medications are usually less expensive, and extended-release forms are available. Disadvantages are that the drugs cannot be given orally to unconscious patients, patients who are ventilated mechanically, or patients who have trouble swallowing. There is also a time delay between administration and the onset of action; and food, other drugs, acid, or lack of acid may interfere with absorption.

Sublingual and Buccal

Both of these routes are administered into the mouth. Sublingual doses are placed under the tongue, while buccal doses are placed inside the cheek. The abbreviation for sublingual is SL. Both of these routes provide rapid onset of action, but buccal is slower than sublingual. *Examples: nitroglycerin (sl), Metandren® linguets (buccal).*

Parenteral

Drugs which are administered via a **parenteral** route bypass the gastrointestinal tract. Drugs administered this way may be given over a short (seconds to minutes) or extended (hours to days) period. These drugs are usually formulated as solutions but may also be emulsions or **suspensions**. *Examples: Intralipid®, Sus-Phrine®.*

The advantages of the parenteral routes are that they can be used in patients who cannot take drugs orally, they have a faster onset of action, and they can be used when the drug is unstable in the acid environment of the stomach. Disadvantages of the parenteral route are the invasive (needle penetrates the skin) nature, it can be very painful, there is a risk of infection, and the drugs are usually more expensive.

The abbreviation for the intravenous route is *IV* because the drug is injected through a needle directly into a vein. The injected solution must be sterile and free of particles. When a caregiver administers a drug by this route, it is immediately available to act in the body, but it may be difficult to reverse the drug effect.

When a drug is given intravenously over a short period, it is called a *bolus* and is described as administered by *IV push* (IVP) via syringe and needle. If the drug is infused into a vein over hours or days by constant infusion or drip, it is described as *IV piggyback* (IVPB). This method provides a continuous supply of the drug to the body.

When a drug is administered by a direct **injection** into large muscle, it is called *intramuscular*, abbreviated IM. The most common sites for intramuscular injections include the upper arm (deltoid muscle), thigh, or buttock. Intramuscular injections may be solutions or suspensions.

The advantages of intramuscular injection include a more rapid onset than oral and extended-release forms. The disadvantages of the intramuscular route are the following:

- It is difficult to reverse.
- It may be painful and cause bruising.
- Absorption may be erratic and incomplete.
- Only a limited volume of drug can be injected.
- It is risky in patients with decreased muscle mass, bleeding disorders, or who are taking anticoagulants.

When a drug is injected under the skin (in fatty tissue), but not directly into a muscle, the route of administration is called *subcutaneous*, abbreviated SC, subQ, or SQ. Drugs administered this way are absorbed more slowly and less completely than by IV or IM routes. Advantages of the subcutaneous route are that patients can be taught to self-administer their doses. The disadvantages include the following:

- Only a limited volume of injection may be given.
- The injection cannot be given into frail skin.
- It should not be given by this route to patients with bleeding disorders or who are receiving anticoagulants (blood thinners).

A few other parenteral routes are listed in the table below:

ROUTE	DESCRIPTION	ABBREVIATION
intradermal	into the top layer of skin	ID
intra-arterial	into an artery	IA
intra-articular	into a joint	
intracardiac	into the heart	IC
intraperitoneal	into the abdominal cavity	
intrapleural	into the sac surrounding the lung	
intraventricular	into the cavities of the brain	
intrathecal	into the space around the spinal cord	
intravaginal	into the vagina	
intraocular	into an eye	

Topical

The **topical** route of administration refers to the application of a drug to the surface of the skin or mucous membranes. Drugs administered this way include creams, ointments, lotions, sprays, aerosols, and powders. This route is used to treat topically (steroids) or may be absorbed into the blood stream (nitroglycerin ointment).

The topical route of administration also includes the **transdermal** route. This route is through the skin and is used to deliver the drug systemically. The drug is contained in an adhesive patch that is applied directly to the skin. *Examples: Duragesic®, Estraderm®, Catapres-TTS®, Habitrol®, Nitro-Dur®.*

Other Routes

The **rectal** route provides access through the anus into the rectum. It is abbreviated PR (*per rectum*). This route is useful for children or if the oral route is unavailable. This route is also useful when treating nausea and vomiting because orally administered medications may be lost when the patient throws up. Drugs administered by the rectal route may provide a local (**enema** for evacuating the bowel) or systemic effect. Examples of drugs administered by this route include solids, solutions, suspensions, or foams. *Examples: Compazine® suppository for nausea, Phenergan® suppository, Fleet® enema solution, barium contrast media suspension, and ProctoFoam®.*

The vaginal route of administration requires that the drug be inserted into the vagina. When given this way, the drug may have local or systemic action. The typical dosage forms administered vaginally include suppository, tablet, cream, ointment, gel, and solution.

Drugs are administered by the **otic** route when they are placed into the ear canal. These dosage forms are formulated as solutions or suspensions. The route is abbreviated as AD (*aura dextro*, right ear), AS (*aura sinister*, left ear), or AU (*aura utro*, both ears).

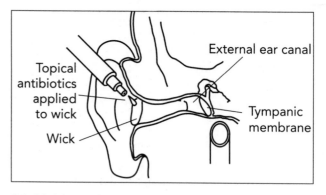

Otic Administration

The **ophthalmic** route of administration is into the eye and is abbreviated OD (oculo *dexter*, right eye), OS (*oculo sinister*, left eye), and OU (*oculos utro*, both eyes). Dosage forms for ophthalmic administration include gels, solutions, suspensions, ointments, and inserts, with the most common being solutions.

The **nasal** route affords access for drug administration into the nostrils via sprays or drops. The drug may provide a local or systemic effect.

Drugs that are administered by **inhalation** enter through the mouth into the lungs. There is a rapid onset of action, and this route is usually used to treat local lung disease such as asthma or systemic disease like the flu. *Examples: Isuprel®, Relenza®.*

Practice Questions

1. Which of the following is/are route(s) of drug administration?
   a. suppository
   b. injection
   c. otic
   d. all of the above

2. When the prescriber's instructions indicate that the patient should take the drug SL, which directions might be included on the prescription label?
   a. Change the patch every 12 hours.
   b. Chew before swallowing.
   c. Place the medication under the tongue as needed.
   d. Use 0.5 mL in 2 mL of normal saline every four hours as needed.

3. A parenteral route of administration is one that bypasses what?
   a. parents
   b. veins
   c. arteries
   d. gastrointestinal tract

4. How should a prescription with the directions "PR PRN" be administered?
   a. to the right eye as needed
   b. to both eyes as needed
   c. as needed
   d. in the rectum as needed

5. The prescriber orders erythromycin OU. Which of the following medications do you dispense?
   a. otic suspension
   b. otic solution
   c. ophthalmic ointment
   d. both a and b

6. Which of the following routes of administration is/are parenteral route(s)?
   a. rectal
   b. PO
   c. buccal
   d. IVPB

7. Advantages of liquid dosage forms include all of the following EXCEPT
   a. they are faster acting.
   b. they have a shorter expiration time.
   c. they are easier to swallow.
   d. there is a flexibility in dosing.

8. Which of the following is NOT an aqueous solution?
   a. douche
   b. enema
   c. elixir
   d. syrup

9. Medication administered by the IV route usually means that the medication is injected directly into what?
   a. a ventricle of the heart
   b. the eye
   c. a vein
   d. a ventricle of the brain

10. The IV route of administration may be advantageous over the oral route for which reason?
    a. There is less chance of bacterial contamination of the bloodstream.
    b. The drug effects are easily reversed if too high a dose is given.
    c. The drug is available to immediately act in the body.
    d. The drug is absorbed from muscle tissue into the bloodstream, which may provide an extended-release effect.

11. Which dosage form would be best for a patient with an ear canal infection?
   a. tablet
   b. capsule
   c. suppository
   d. suspension

12. Lozenges are also known as
   a. tablets.
   b. troches.
   c. pastilles.
   d. all of the above.

13. How could you interpret AU written on a prescription?
   a. of each
   b. affected area
   c. each ear
   d. each eye

14. The advantages to delivering medications via syringe infusion include which of the following?
   a. Syringes are easy to fill in batches.
   b. Syringes require less storage space.
   c. The drugs stored in syringes are stable for longer.
   d. both a and b

15. Injection of a drug into a muscle is known as what route of medication administration?
   a. ID
   b. SC
   c. IM
   d. IC

16. For which of the following situations would a liquid medication dosage form be a better choice than a solid one?
   a. A patient has just had throat surgery and cannot easily swallow.
   b. A patient is very sensitive to unpleasant tastes and refuses to take "bad-tasting" medicine.
   c. A traveling salesman needs to take a medication on a regular basis.
   d. A patient must take a medication that must be dosed very precisely.

17. Drugs that are administered into the eye are given by what route?
   a. otic
   b. ophthalmic
   c. oral
   d. aural

18. Drugs that are administered into the ear are given by what route?
   a. otic
   b. ophthalmic
   c. oral
   d. buccal

19. Which of the following is not a drug dosage form?
   a. tablet
   b. solution
   c. concoction
   d. injection

20. What do drug formulation aids include?
   a. excipients
   b. preservatives
   c. diluents
   d. all of the above

21. What is a soluble substance called?
   a. solvent
   b. solubilizer
   c. solute
   d. none of the above

22. Which of the following is not a solid dosage form?
   a. capsule
   b. powder
   c. suspension
   d. granule

23. What is the most prescribed ocular dosage form?
   a. eye drops solution
   b. drug-presoaked hydrogel-type contact lens
   c. ocular inserts
   d. core reservoirs in lipophilic membranes

24. What are the advantages of transdermal patches?
   a. convenience
   b. uninterrupted therapy
   c. better patient compliance
   d. all of the above

25. Which of the following statements about medicinal aerosols is correct?
   a. They are slowly dissolved in the mouth.
   b. They are implanted subcutaneously.
   c. They are applied to the skin.
   d. They are inhaled through nose or mouth.

26. Which of the following statements about trans-dermal patches is correct?
   a. They are slowly dissolved in the mouth.
   b. They are implanted subcutaneously.
   c. They are applied to the skin.
   d. They are inhaled through nose or mouth.

27. Lozenges are
   a. slowly dissolved in the mouth.
   b. implanted subcutaneously.
   c. applied to the skin.
   d. inhaled through nose or mouth.

28. Pellets are
   a. slowly dissolved in the mouth.
   b. implanted subcutaneously.
   c. applied to the skin.
   d. inhaled through nose or mouth.

29. What is the range of capsule sizes?
   a. from,000 (smallest) to 5 (largest)
   b. from,000 (largest) to 5 (smallest)
   c. from 0 (smallest) to 5 (largest)
   d. from 0 (largest) to 5 (smallest)

30. What is a drug dosage form that consists of a high concentration of a sugar in water called?
   a. solution
   b. spirit
   c. syrup
   d. aromatic water

31. Medication dosage forms include
   a. liquids.
   b. semisolids.
   c. gases.
   d. all of the above.

32. What is the safest and most convenient route of drug administration?
   a. rectal
   b. inhalation
   c. oral
   d. parenteral

33. The mucous membrane is a route of administration for all of the following EXCEPT
   a. transdermal patches.
   b. inhalation.
   c. suppositories.
   d. troches.

34. Which dosage forms are appropriate for the
vaginal route of administration?
   a. suppositories and tablets
   b. fluid solutions and creams
   c. foams
   d. all of the above

35. The rectal route of administration is useful if
the patient is
   a. nauseated.
   b. vomiting.
   c. unconscious.
   d. all of the above.

36. Extended-release tablets or capsules should
not be
   a. chewed.
   b. cut.
   c. dissolved in liquid.
   d. all of the above.

37. Subcutaneous injections are given
   a. in the muscle.
   b. outside the spinal cord.
   c. into the fatty tissue.
   d. none of the above

38. Which of the following statements is false?
   a. Suspensions are used for drugs that are not
   readily soluble (able to dissolve).
   b. Extended-release dosage forms are
   commonly referred to as *long-acting*.
   c. Tablets never include inert (inactive)
   ingredients.
   d. all of the above

39. Which of the following types of injections is
inserted just below the surface of the skin?
   a. intramuscular
   b. intradermal
   c. intracardiac
   d. subcutaneous

40. Of the following drugs, which one would you
not want to crush and put in applesauce to
make it easier to swallow?
   a. Bayer® aspirin
   b. Entex LA®
   c. Tylenol®
   d. codeine

Answers and Explanations

1. c. Otic is the route of drug administration; suppository and injection are dosage forms.

2. c. SL is the abbreviation for sublingual, or under the tongue.

3. d. A parenteral route of administration is one that bypasses the gastrointestinal tract, which is referred to as an enteral route of administration.

4. d. The directions PR PRN refer to *in the rectum as needed*; PR stands for *per rectum* and PRN for *as needed*. The eye is the ophthalmic route.

5. c. This medication is ophthalmic ointment; OU means both eyes; otic is signified by the abbreviation AU, AD, or AS. Medications placed into the eye must be sterile to prevent infection, and ear drops are not sterile.

6. d. The parenteral route of administration is IVPB. This abbreviation stands for *intravenous piggyback*, which is a way of introducing drugs through an already running IV line.

7. b. A shorter expiration time is not an advantage of liquid dosage forms because the drug is dissolved in an aqueous phase, and its stability is reduced.

8. c. An elixir is a hydro-alcoholic solution; all the others are aqueous.

9. c. When medication is administered by the IV route, it is usually injected directly into a vein.

10. c. The IV route of administration may be advantageous over the oral route because the drug is available to act immediately in the body. Drugs given via an IV are already dissolved, bypass the gastrointestinal system, and do not rely on blood flow to the muscle for absorption.

11. d. Suspension is the best dosage form for a patient with an ear canal infection, as the other dosage forms are inappropriate or impossible to use in the ear.

12. d. Lozenges are also known as tablets, troches, and pastilles.

13. c. The prescription abbreviation AU stands for both ears, AA means *of each* or *affected area*, and OU means *each eye*.

14. d. The advantages to delivering medications via syringe infusion are that syringes are easy to fill in batches, and they require less storage. However, drugs are less stable when repackaged into a syringe.

15. c. Injection of a drug into a muscle is known as an *intramuscular*, or IM, route of medication administration. *Intradermal*, or ID, would be just underneath the skin; *subcutaneous*, or SC, would be in the fatty tissue under the skin; and *intracardiac*, or IC, would be an injection into the heart.

16. a. A patient who has just had throat surgery and cannot swallow easily should be given a liquid medication dosage. Liquid dosage forms enhance an unpleasant taste, are more bulky than solid dosage forms and are therefore inconvenient when traveling, and solid dosage forms are dosed much more precisely than liquids can be measured.

17. b. Drugs that are administered into the eye are given by the ophthalmic route.

18. a. Drugs that are administered into the ear are given by the otic route.

19. c. A concoction is a combination of various ingredients—usually herbs, spices, condiments, powdery substances, or minerals mixed together, minced, dissolved, or macerated into a liquid to be ingested.

20. d. Excipients, preservatives, and diluents are all drug formulation aids.

21. c. A soluble substance is called a solute. A solvent is the liquid in which a solute dissolves, and a solubilizer enhances the dissolution of another substance in a solvent.

22. c. A suspension is a liquid dosage form in which undissolved particles float.

23. a. The most prescribed ocular dosage form is eye drops (solution).

24. d. Convenience, uninterrupted therapy, and better patient compliance are all advantages of transdermal patches.

25. d. Medicinal aerosols are inhaled through nose or mouth. Troches, pastilles, lozenges, and buccal and sublingual tablets are slowly dissolved in the mouth; pills are implanted subcutaneously; and ointments, creams, and patches are applied to the skin.

26. c. Transdermal patches are applied to the skin (as are ointments and creams). Medicinal aerosols are inhaled through the nose or mouth. Troches, pastilles, lozenges, and buccal and sublingual tablets are slowly dissolved in the mouth, and pills are implanted subcutaneously.

27. a. Lozenges are slowly dissolved in the mouth (as are troches, pastilles, and buccal and sublingual tablets). Medicinal aerosols are inhaled through nose or mouth. Pills are implanted subcutaneously, and ointments, creams, and patches are applied to the skin.

28. b. Pellets are implanted subcutaneously (as are pills). Medicinal aerosols are inhaled through the nose or mouth. Troches, pastilles, lozenges, and buccal and sublingual tablets are slowly dissolved in the mouth, and ointments, creams, and patches are applied to the skin.

29. b. Capsule sizes range from,000 (largest) to 5 (smallest).

30. c. A drug dosage form that consists of a high concentration of a sugar in water is called a syrup. A solution may or may not contain sugar, a spirit contains alcohol and may or may not contain sugar, and an aromatic water is a mixture of water with a volatile oil.

31. d. Liquids, semisolids, and gases are all medication dosage forms. Gaseous dosage forms include inhalation anesthetics.

32. c. The safest and most convenient route of drug administration is oral. Rectal is less convenient than oral, and inhalational and parenteral routes are difficult to reverse if there is an adverse reaction to the drug.

33. a. The mucous membrane is not a route of administration for transdermal patches. Transdermal patches should be applied only to unbroken skin with minimal hair present.

34. d. Suppositories and tablets, fluid solutions and creams, and foams are all appropriate dosage forms for the vaginal route of administration. Foams include anti-inflammatory agents and contraceptives; douches are fluid solutions and are used to treat local infections as are tablets, creams, and suppositories.

35. d. If the patient is nauseated, vomiting, or unconscious, the rectal route of administration is useful. No medication should be administered orally to an unconscious patient; medications given to someone who is nauseated or vomiting have a high probability of not being retained long enough to produce a therapeutic effect.

36. d. Extended-release capsules should not be chewed, crushed, cut, or dissolved in any liquid, as this will release the full strength of the drug at one time.

37. c. Subcutaneous injections are given in the fatty tissue beneath the last layer of skin. Injection in the muscle would be IM, injections surrounding the spinal cord are intrathecal or epidural.

38. c. Tablets must contain inert (inactive) ingredients. These would include binders, diluents, lubricants, colors, disintegrators, sweeteners, and flavors.

39. b. Injection just below the surface of the skin is called an *intradermal*, or ID, injection.

40. b. The abbreviation LA following the drug name means long-acting, which tells you that you should not crush this tablet. By crushing this tablet, you will have the whole 12-hour strength of medication at once instead of slow delivery over a 12-hour period, as intended. The other medications may be crushed and placed in applesauce if needed, as they are not long-acting or sustained-release.

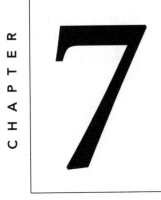

7 ▶ Basic Anatomy and Physiology

CHAPTER OVERVIEW

When we talk about drug therapy in a basic sense, it is necessary to learn and understand anatomy (structures), physiology (function), specific disease states, mechanisms of drug action, and the effects of specific drugs on the human body as well. This chapter will give you a basic overview that should allow you to understand more precise content in the following chapters.

KEY TERMS

adverse reaction

anatomy

arteries

atrium

blood

bone marrow

bones

brain

capillaries

cardiac muscle

central nervous system

dermis

drug classification

endocrine system

epidermis

gastrointestinal system

heart

indication

integumentary system

ovaries

pancreas

pathology

pharmacodynamics

pharmacokinetics

physiology

respiratory system

sebaceous gland

sebum

skeletal muscle

smooth muscle

somatic nervous system

spinal cord

subcutaneous layer

sweat gland

testes

thyroid gland

veins

ventricle

Anatomy and Physiology Overview

Anatomy is the study of the different structures of the body and how they are organized. **Physiology** is the study of the functions of these body parts, what they do, and how they do it. There are also what we call different *body systems*, which coordinate with each other to help the body maintain homeostasis (or equilibrium).

Following are examples of body systems, as well as some diseases and conditions associated with those body systems.

The Integumentary System

The **integumentary system**, also referred to as the skin and its appendages (such as hair and nails), acts as a physical barrier between the external environment and the internal structures of the body. The integumentary system helps thermoregulation (regulating body temperature) through sweat glands and muscles attached to the hair follicles.

Epidermis is the outermost layer of the skin. This layer contains the melanocytes, which is where the pigment is stored. Pigment expresses the coloration of the skin. Although the skin acts as a barrier to the outside world, the process of keratinization causes the new skin cells to put older ones on the surface, where they change shape and composition, die, and are replaced. These dead skin cells help protect against pathogens that may otherwise be able to penetrate the skin.

Dermis is the middle layer of the skin and is often referred to as the "true skin." It contains fibroblasts, which secrete elastin, collagen, and ground substance. Fibroblasts are responsible for providing support and elasticity of the skin. Other vital structures found in this layer include immune cells, hair follicles, sweat and oil glands, and sensory receptors.

The **subcutaneous layer** is the innermost portion of the skin. It is made up of adipose, which is fat and connective tissue. This layer helps to protect against heat, UV rays, and infection.

Sweat Glands

The **sweat gland** is a two-part gland that consists of a secretory portion and an excretory duct. The secretory portion is located below the dermis and produces the sweat. The excretory duct spirals through the dermis and exits at the surface of the skin. Sweating releases moisture that evaporates and cools the body. There are between two and four million sweat glands in the human body.

Sebaceous Glands

The **sebaceous gland** forms along the sides of the walls of the hair follicle and produces **sebum**. Sebum is an oily substance responsible for lubricating the skin. It is controlled by the **endocrine system**.

Functions of the Skin

There are four main functions of the skin: sensation, protection, heat regulation, and secretion.

Sensation occurs when receptor sites can detect changes in external temperature and pressure. Protection prevents the passage of harmful physical and chemical agents. Heat regulation allows the body to adjust temperature by using the muscles that surround hair follicles and sweat glands. The skin secretes sebum, which has anti-fungal and antibacterial properties, and sweat, which cools the body.

Diseases and Conditions of the Integumentary System

- rash: an area of red, inflamed skin
- bacterial infection: occurs when bacteria lies on the surface of the skin
- viral infection: occurs when a virus penetrates the skin
- parasitic infection: occurs when a worm or insect burrows into the skin to live or lay eggs
- fungal infection: occurs when a fungus gains entry to the skin

The Nervous System

The nervous system is made up of both the central and peripheral nervous systems. The function of the nervous system is to direct the voluntary or involuntary actions of the body. It does so by sending electrical messages to and from the **brain**.

Central Nervous System

The **central nervous system** (CNS) contains the brain and **spinal cord**. Messages are sent up the spinal cord from sensory receptors, where they are processed and interpreted by the brain. Once this done, the brain can send a response. For example, an increase in body temperature will cause the brain to signal the sweat glands to secrete sweat.

The peripheral nervous system (PNS) contains nerves that branch out from the central nervous system to body limbs and organs. These nerves receive responses from the brain to allow functions of the body to occur, such as limb movement, and also send external stimuli back to the central nervous system.

The Brain

The brain is protected by the skull and three layers of membrane called the meninges. It is responsible for receiving and interpreting stimuli and sending messages back to motor structures, which act on the stimuli.

The brain is divided into four lobes:

- frontal lobe
- parietal lobe
- temporal lobe
- occipital lobe

The largest part of the brain is the cerebrum, which is divided into two parts—the cerebral cortex and the cerebral medulla.

Spinal Cord

The other significant part of the CNS is the spinal cord: a long, thin, tubular bundle of nervous tissues that extends from the brain down the backbone and to all parts of the body. It functions to transmit neural signals to and from the brain and other parts of the body.

The Nervous System's Effect on Body Systems

The nervous system has an effect on each body system to ensure homeostasis, or equilibrium. As the nervous system continually monitors the body systems, it can adjust the systems' production based on its needs.

The integumentary system is affected by the brain, as sensory receptors send information about the external environment.

The cardiovascular system is affected, as baroreceptors send information to the brain about blood pressure. The nervous system responds by causing vessels to constrict or dilate.

For the respiratory system, the brain monitors respiratory volume and blood gas levels. It then responds to these values by regulating respiratory rate.

The gastrointestinal system is in control of movement of the digestive tract. The nervous system also controls feelings of thirst and hunger.

The brain controls the muscular system through its movement of skeletal muscle and regulation of heart rate.

For the skeletal system, sensory receptors in the bones and joints send signals about the body's position to the brain. The skull and vertebrae also protect the brain and spinal cord from injury.

The hypothalamus in the brain also affects the endocrine system, as it controls all endocrine glands.

The immune system is also impacted, as the brain stimulates the defense mechanisms that fight off pathogens.

Some Diseases and Conditions of the Nervous System

- Anxiety: A feeling of uneasiness, apprehension, fear, and worry that affects an individual ability to function normally. This can be acute (short period of time) or chronic, lasting a long period of time. Though not fully understood, neurotransmitters (messengers of the brain) seem to play a role.
- Depression: Constant feelings of sadness, irritability, and lack of concentration. This may be

acute (short period of time) or chronic (lasting a long period of time). Though not fully understood, neurotransmitters (messengers of the brain) seem to play a role.

- Bipolar disorder or manic depression: Characterized by peaks of extreme emotional highs and lows that can span days, weeks, or months.
- Seizures: Characterized by convulsions or involuntary muscle movements of the body caused by irregular electrical activity in the brain. Type of seizure is dependent on where the focus (origin) of electrical activity occurs.
- Parkinson's disease: Symptoms include, but are not limited to, tremor, stiffness, and slowing of movement. Involvement of the neurotransmitter dopamine (too little) seems to play a role in this disease state.
- Schizophrenia: Characterized by abnormalities in a patient's perception or expression of reality. Involvement of the neurotransmitter dopamine (too much) seems to play a role in this disease state.

The Cardiovascular System

The cardiovascular system consists of the heart and the vessels that carry blood to and from the heart. This system works in tandem with the respiratory system to carry oxygen to all parts of the body, while carrying away carbon dioxide and waste, which are harmful to cells.

The Heart

The heart is divided into left and right sides, each containing an **atrium**—the top chamber—and **ventricle**—the bottom chamber. The heart is made up of myocardium, also known as cardiac muscle, which provides the contractions needed to pump the **blood** out of the heart.

Arteries

Arteries are vessels that carry oxygen-rich blood away from the heart and toward all the tissues, cells, and organs in the body.

Veins

Veins are vessels that carry oxygen-depleted blood toward the heart so that it can be pumped to the lungs to replenish its supply of oxygen.

Capillaries

Capillaries are the smallest of the body's vessels, only one cell thick. Although small, the capillaries allow the exchange of water, oxygen, carbon dioxide, nutrients, and waste between the blood and the surrounding tissues.

Blood

Blood is a liquid tissue that is responsible for life, growth, and health. An average person has approximately 5.6 liters of blood in his or her body. It serves as an effective transport system for oxygen, nutrients, disease-fighting cells, and hormones.

Diseases of the Cardiovascular System

- coronary artery disease (CAD): narrowing of the vessels that supply blood to the heart
- hypertension: high blood pressure
- arrhythmia: irregular heart beat
- thrombosis: formation of a blood clot
- myocardial infarction (MI): also known as a heart attack, it is the heart's response to a lack of oxygen
- stroke: a clot that travels to the brain and blocks the flow of oxygen to it

The Respiratory System

The **respiratory system** includes the organs responsible for exchanging carbon dioxide for air—a collection of gases, including oxygen. Oxygen is needed so the body can convert nutrients gained from food into a usable form of energy. The respiratory system is divided into two parts: the upper and lower repiratory tracts.

Upper Respiratory Tract

This is the place where the air enters the respiratory system and is filtered and warmed before it is passed into the lower respiratory tract. This part of the system includes the mouth, nose, sinuses, and larynx.

Lower Respiratory Tract

This is where the air is taken into the body so it can be carried to all tissues. It includes the trachea, bronchi, bronchioles, alveoli, and lungs. The trachea, bronchi, and bronchioles lead to the alveoli, which are tiny air sacs surrounded by capillaries. These allow the air to enter into the bloodstream.

Some Diseases and Conditions of the Respiratory System

- bronchitis: inflammation of the bronchial tubes
- emphysema: destruction of the air sacs found in the lungs
- upper respiratory infection: viral or bacterial infection concentrated in the mouth, nose, sinuses, and larynx
- asthma: narrowing of the airway caused by an irritant
- cystic fibrosis: a condition that causes the formation of thick, sticky mucus

The Gastrointestinal System

The **gastrointestinal system** is a series of hollow tubes for digestion that run from the mouth down through the body to the anus. The digestive process has five stages: ingestion, digestion, movement, absorption, and elimination. The main organs of the digestive system are the mouth, pharynx, esophagus, stomach, and small and large intestines.

Mouth

The mouth is the site of physical food breakdown. The teeth help to create greater surface area by breaking down large pieces into smaller ones. The tongue moves the food around the mouth, allowing the teeth to work more efficiently. Meanwhile, the saliva glands secrete liquids to aid in digestion.

Esophagus

The esophagus is a tube that connects the mouth and stomach. At the end of the esophagus is a circular muscle, called the cardiac sphincter, which prevents the acid inside of the stomach from splashing up and damaging the esophagus.

Stomach

The stomach is a saclike organ where chemical breakdown takes place. It secretes hydrochloric acid that breaks down the ingested food so it can begin to be absorbed by the small intestine. As the stomach is taking in food, it will work in two parts for effective digestion. The first part is a staging, or holding, area, which is near the fundus. As the food moves toward the pylorus, that part of the stomach churns the food inside the acid, allowing for faster chemical breakdown.

Small Intestine

Food exits the stomach and moves into into the small intestine. A circular muscle, similar to the one at the top of the stomach, called the pyloric sphincter, separates the stomach and the small intestine. This is where the absorption of nutrients and medications takes place. The **pancreas** and liver aid this process by secreting enzymes, allowing the breakdown and absorption of nutrients to continue as they pass through the small intestine. Anything not absorbed by the small intestine is passed on as waste.

Large Intestine

This organ is responsible for eliminating the waste passed on by the small intestine. As the waste moves through the large intestine, the solid is separated from the liquid so it can reabsorb water back into the body to prevent dehydration. The large intestine is separated into seven parts: cecum, asending colon, transverse colon, descending colon, sigmoid colon, rectum, and anus.

Some Diseases and Conditions of the Gastrointestinal System

- gastroesophageal reflux disease (GERD): caused when acid from the stomach splashes onto the esophagus
- nausea and vomiting: the awareness that something is stimulating the vomit center in the brain followed by the involuntary contraction of the abdominal muscles
- H. pylori: a bacterial infection in the mucosa that causes an increase in acid production
- ulcer: a sore that forms in the stomach or small intestine commonly caused by an excess production of stomach acid
- ulcerative colitis: an inflammation of the large intestine and rectum

The Musculoskeletal System

The musculoskeletal system includes the combination of the muscles and bones, which provide the body with support and allow both voluntary and involuntary movement.

Muscles

There are three types of muscles throughout the body: skeletal, smooth, and cardiac. These muscles provide the body with its ability to generate movement.

- The skeletal muscle is a voluntary muscle that pulls on the bones, allowing movement. The muscles are connected to the bones by tendons.
- The **smooth muscle** is an involuntary muscle that either pushes blood through vessels or food through intestines. It is controlled by the autonomic portion of the peripheral nervous system.
- The **cardiac muscle** is also involuntary and found exclusively in the **heart**. It is responsible for generating electrical stimulation and contractions necessary for pumping blood.

Bones

Bones provide support and protection for the body. They are made up of dense connective tissue infused with a calcified substance. As adults, we have 206 bones in our body, each containing marrow inside of them. Another important function of the bones is to protect vital organs from injury. The best example is the ribcage, protecting the heart and lungs.

Bone marrow is a gelatinous substance found inside bones. Red marrow is responsible for producing red blood cells, white blood cells, and platelets. Yellow marrow, which is found in most bones at the onset of adulthood, is used for fat storage.

Diseases and Conditions of the Musculoskeletal System

- osteomyelitis: infection of the bone
- osteoporosis: a loss of bone density, which causes them to become brittle
- arthritis: inflammation of the joint
- rheumatoid arthritis (RA): autoimmune disease causing pain and inflammation of the joint
- tendonitis: inflammation of the tendons
- muscle spasm: the uncontrolled contraction of a muscle

The Endocrine System

The endocrine system is a collection of organs which secrete hormones. It helps to regulate many of the body's functions as it communicates for the nervous system.

Hypothalamus

The hypothalamus is a gland found in the brain which is responsible for releasing hormones that signal the pituitary gland.

Pituitary Gland

The pituitary gland controls the other endocrine organs. It secretes specific hormones that stimulate individual glands, which in turn secrete the hormone that affects change in the body.

Thyroid Gland

The **thyroid gland** is found in the front of the neck and is responsible for metabolism, growth, and body heat production (also known as thermogenesis). The thyroid gland uses iodine to produce the hormones T4 and T3 to regulate the functions mentioned above.

Adrenal Glands

There is an adrenal gland that sits atop each kidney. Besides secreting epinephrine, they are responsible for secreting glucocorticoids and mineralocorticoids. Glucocorticoids are commonly known as anti-stress steroids because they have anti-inflammatory and immunosuppressive properties. Mineralocorticoids are responsible for regulating the salt/water metabolism, which affects blood pressure.

Pancreas

Located in the abdominal cavity below the stomach, the pancreas is responsible for regulating blood glucose levels. In order to properly regulate glucose, the pancreas secretes either glucagon or insulin. Glucagon is the hormone that raises the blood glucose level by converting glycogen into glucose, while insulin is the hormone that lowers the blood glucose level by converting glucose into glycogen.

Some Diseases and Conditions of the Endocrine System

- diabetes: caused by the body's resistance or inability to produce insulin
- hypothyroidism: occurs when the thyroid gland does not produce adequate thyroid hormone
- menopause: caused by the stop in production of female sex hormones
- polycystic ovarian syndrome (PCOS): caused by an excess amount of male hormone
- growth disorders: can be caused by an excess or deficiency in growth hormone

The Reproductive System

The reproductive system's main involvement is in the production of offspring. Other systems, such as the endocrine and circulatory systems, mainly maintain homeostasis for survival purposes, but this system ensures survival of a species. The reproductive system has four functions:

- to produce ova (eggs) and sperm cells
- to transport and sustain these cells
- to nurture the developing offspring
- to produce hormones

Gonads

Gonads, which are also considered part of the endocrine system, are sex-specific organs that secrete hormones responsible for secondary sex characteristics and reproduction. In males, these organs are the **testes**. In females, they are the **ovaries**.

Testes are found, outside the body, in the scrotum. They are responsible for the production of androgens, which stimulate the development of the sex organs and defining characteristics. Also produced in the testes is sperm—the male sex cell responsible for reproduction.

Ovaries are found in the pelvic cavity. They are responsible for the production of estrogens and progesterones. Estrogen is responsible for the development of secondary sexual characteristics while progesterone is responsible for stimulating the uterine lining for fertilization. The egg, which is the female sex cell, is also found in the ovaries.

Some Diseases and Conditions of the Reproductive System

- herpes: viral infection that produces sores on the genitals
- chlamydia: bacterial infection in the reproductive tract
- genital warts: infection that causes wartlike bumps on the genitals

- gonorrhea: bacterial infection in the reproductive tract
- HIV/AIDS: viral infection that affects the immune system

The Immune System

The immune system is responsible for protecting the body against pathogens and foreign material. It does so by using one of two protection methods—specific and nonspecific defense mechanisms.

Nonspecific Defense Mechanisms

These mechanisms indicate that the protection method is not specific to the pathogen or foreign material. Some examples of nonspecific defense mechanisms include mucus in the respiratory tract that traps particles, tears that flush out irritants from the eyes, and clotting that prevents pathogens from entering the bloodstream.

Specific Defense Mechanisms

These defense mechanisms are specific to individual pathogens and are commonly referred to as antibodies. The most common specific defense mechanisms are T-cells and B-cells.

B-cells form in the liver and contain one inserted antibody. As it enters the bloodstream, it will multiply to protect against the same pathogen. Once a B-cell attaches to a pathogen, it will either become a plasma or memory cell.

T-cells are formed right before and after birth. They develop in the thymus gland and reside in the lymph nodes. They provide a resistance to specific disease-causing agents.

Terms Found in the Healthcare Profession

Pathology

Pathology is the study and diagnosis of disease and its processes. The basic understanding of pathology will allow pharmacy technicians a better understanding of disease states and mechanism of drug action (MOA) as well. Below are the most common diseases found in each body system.

Types of Pathogens

Pathogens are microorganisms that cause disease. The following are the most common sources of pathogens.

- Animal microorganisms are commonly parasites that are bacterial, protozoal, or worm. The bacterial and protozoal microorganisms are single-celled disease-causing agents, while worms are multicellular.
- Viruses are infectious agents that can only replicate inside a host cell.
- Autoimmune diseases occur when the body becomes the target of its own defenses. The body's immune system essentially thinks that its own cells, tissues, and/or organs are pathogens.
- Plant microorganisms are single-celled organisms that secrete digestive enzymes onto the organic molecules they are living on so they can feed on the dying cells. These include fungi, yeast, and mold.
- Prions are pathogens that are only made of protein. These are disease-causing agents that typically affect the brain. Prions cause diseases like mad cow disease.

Susceptible Host

A susceptible host refers to a person who has little or no immunity to infection and has been infected by a pathogen.

Pharmacology

Pharmacology is the study of the interactions between living organisms and medications. Although it is not a topic of focus for the national exam, a basic knowledge of pharmacology does give the pharmacy technician a better understanding of his or her role in the pharmacy setting. In addition to knowing brand and generic names, main indications, and drug classifications, a basic understanding of mechanism of drug action is necessary as well.

Pharmacokinetics

Pharmacokinetics is the study of absorption, distribution, metabolism, and excretion of a drug in the body, or how a drug moves and changes when introduced into the body. Pharmacokinetics is important in that the dosing of medications need to be as exact as possible, especially in the hospital setting. Clinical pharmacists will generally do pharmacokinetics for physicians and recommend doses of medication to be given. In some cases, pharmacy technicians help the clinical pharmacist in collecting necessary data.

Drug Agonist

A drug agonist is a drug that will cause a reaction to occur in the body. In the case of the drug albuterol (brand name Ventolin®), the drug will relax the smooth muscles of the bronchioles, thus causing relaxation and opening of the bronchioles for easy breathing.

Drug Antagonist

Drug antagonist is a drug that will cause a reaction not to occur or block a reaction from occurring. An example would be an antihistamine such as Benadryl® or diphenhydramine HCl, which will block histamine 1 receptor sites from stimulation by the endogenous compound histamine. By blocking stimulation, an allergic reaction will not occur.

Pharmacodynamics

Pharmacodynamics is the study of the physiological effects a medication has on the body or microorganisms within the body. This is vital to our understanding of the mechanism of action and **adverse reactions**.

Mechanism of Action

Mechanism of action is how the medication produces a pharmacological effect. For example, an ACE inhibitor reduces blood pressure by inhibiting the conversion of the angiotensin I enzyme into an angiotensin II enzyme, which is a natural vasoconstrictor.

Drug-Drug Interactions

Drug-drug interactions occur when one drug prevents another drug from having the therapeutic (wanted) effect. If this occurs, one or both medications could potentially exacerbate the condition being treated, damage the body, or kill the patient.

Drug-Food Interactions

Drug-food interactions occur when a medication interacts with one or more of the chemicals found in food. This can lead to decreased absorption, increased plasma concentration levels, or an increased release of chemicals by the body.

Indication

Indication, or use, is described as an approved usage for a medication to treat a disease or condition. The governing body which classifies indications is the FDA. Medications can also have "off-label uses," which are treatments for diseases, but are not FDA-approved.

Drug Classification

Drug classification is defined as a group of medications with the same or similar characteristics. These medications can treat or cure the same disease and have similar chemical structure, MOA, and side/adverse effects associated with them.

Adverse Reaction

An adverse reaction, or side effect, is defined as harmful or undesired effects resulting from the use of a medication. Although a medication may have many side effects, a patient may experience some or none of them. In addition, these side effects may subside after a short duration of continued use.

Practice Questions

1. Which of the following is a function of the skin?
   a. secretes hormones
   b. acts as a barrier
   c. releases digestive enzymes
   d. none of the above

2. What organ is responsible for producing sperm in males?
   a. ovaries
   b. testes
   c. pancreas
   d. thyroid

3. Which condition is characterized as a sore that forms in the stomach or small intestine?
   a. colitis
   b. GERD
   c. ulcer
   d. H. pylori

4. Which of the following is another term for external exchange?
   a. blood pressure
   b. respiration
   c. nerve impulse
   d. immune defense

5. Which of the following is an infection in the bone?
   a. arthritis
   b. osteoporosis
   c. osteomyelitis
   d. tendonitis

6. What is the study of the structures of the body?
   a. anatomy
   b. pathology
   c. phrenology
   d. scientology

7. Which gland or glands are responsible for controlling all endocrine glands?
   a. hypothalamus-pituitary
   b. thyroid
   c. pancreas
   d. adrenal

8. Which of the following actions does the nervous system control?
   a. involuntary
   b. indirect
   c. voluntary
   d. both a and c

9. What is the study of the functions of the body parts?
   a. scientology
   b. reflexology
   c. kinesiology
   d. physiology

10. Which gland controls the metabolism of the body?
    a. thyroid
    b. thymus
    c. adrenal
    d. pituitary

11. Which muscle provides the contractions of the heart needed to pump blood?
    a. smooth muscle
    b. skeletal muscle
    c. pericardium
    d. cardiac muscle

12. Which of the following is a vessel that carries oxygen-rich blood to the body?
    a. vein
    b. atrium
    c. artery
    d. vena cava

13. Which organ is found in the pelvic cavity?
 a. liver
 b. stomach
 c. thyroid
 d. ovaries

14. Which of the following refers to the general or common name of a medication?
 a. generic name
 b. brand name
 c. trade name
 d. propriety name

15. The large intestine is responsible for which of the following functions?
 a. the reabsorption of water
 b. the absorption of nutrients
 c. the chemical breakdown
 d. the release of sodium bicarbonate

16. The stomach is responsible for which of the following functions?
 a. physical breakdown
 b. chemical breakdown
 c. absorption of nutrients
 d. excretion

17. Insulin is secreted by which endocrine gland?
 a. pancreas
 b. thyroid
 c. pituitary
 d. testes

18. Which of the following diseases is defined as the body's resistance or inability to produce insulin?
 a. hypothyroidism
 b. diabetes
 c. polycystic ovarian syndrome
 d. growth disorder

19. Which of the following is defined as the study of how a drug moves and changes when introduced into the body?
 a. pharmacodynamics
 b. mechanism of action
 c. indication
 d. pharmacokinetics

20. Which of the following is an inflammation of the bronchial tubes?
 a. emphysema
 b. bronchitis
 c. URI
 d. cystic fibrosis

21. The main function of the small intestines is the
 a. chemical breakdown of food.
 b. reabsorption of water.
 c. absorption of nutrients.
 d. physical breakdown of food.

22. Which gland is responsible for secreting the anti-stress hormone, glucocorticoid?
 a. thyroid gland
 b. adrenal gland
 c. pancreas
 d. gonads

23. The hormones secreted by the endocrine system send messages for which other organ system?
 a. cardiovascular system
 b. nervous system
 c. gastrointestinal system
 d. musculoskeletal system

24. Red marrow gives rise to
 a. white blood cells.
 b. red blood cells.
 c. platelets.
 d. all of the above.

25. Which condition occurs when a clot travels to the brain, blocking the flow of oxygen?
  a. CAD
  b. myocardial infarction
  c. hypertension
  d. stroke

26. Which condition is characterized as an area of red, inflamed skin?
  a. rash
  b. viral infection
  c. bacterial infection
  d. fungal infection

27. Which of the following is defined as the study of the physiological effects that medication has on the body?
  a. pharmacodynamics
  b. metabolism
  c. absorption
  d. pharmacokinetics

28. Which of the following conditions would be associated with the symptoms of constant sadness, irritability, and lack of concentration?
  a. seizures
  b. depression
  c. schizophrenia
  d. anxiety

29. The central nervous system contains
  a. motor structures.
  b. sensory receptors.
  c. the spinal cord.
  d. the autonomic system.

30. How many bones are in an adult human body?
  a. 300
  b. 267
  c. 206
  d. 500

31. Hypertension is also known as
  a. stroke.
  b. heart attack.
  c. arrhythmia.
  d. high blood pressure.

32. Parkinson's disease occurs due to the lack of which neurotransmitter?
  a. dopamine
  b. serotonin
  c. endorphin
  d. monoamines

33. CAD restricts blood flow to the heart, which can cause which of the following?
  a. migraines
  b. myocardial infarction
  c. atrial flutter
  d. AV node

34. What are the top chambers of the heart called?
  a. atria
  b. ventricles
  c. mitral valves
  d. aortic valves

35. Which of the following is also referred to as the medication's use?
  a. action
  b. classification
  c. indication
  d. interaction

36. What is a group of medications with similar characteristics called?
  a. generics
  b. drug classification
  c. indication
  d. action

37. Which of the following is defined as a loss of bone density?
   a. osteomyelitis
   b. osteoporosis
   c. arthritis
   d. tendonitis

38. How many chambers does the human heart have?
   a. one
   b. two
   c. three
   d. four

39. What is known as an undesired effect resulting from the use of a medication?
   a. interaction
   b. indication
   c. adverse reaction
   d. action

40. Pharmacokinetics is important in the dosing of medications that need to be as exact as possible, such as in the hospital setting.
   a. true
   b. false

Answers and Explanations

1. b. The skin is a barrier between the outside world and the internal environment. The endocrine system secretes hormones, and the gastrointestinal tract releases digestive enzymes.

2. b. The testes are the only endocrine organ listed that produces sperm. Ovaries are responsible for releasing eggs in females, the pancreas is responsible for secreting insulin, and the thyroid is responsible for secreting T4 and T3 hormone.

3. c. Ulcers are the sores found in the stomach or small intestine. Colitis is inflammation of the bowels; GERD is the erosion of the esophagus; H. pylori is a bacteria.

4. b. The external exchange of gases is respiration.

5. c. Osteomyelitis is a bone infection. Arthritis is inflammation, osteoporosis is the breakdown of bone, and tendonitis is the inflammation of the tendon.

6. a. The study of the structures of the body is anatomy. Pathology is the study of pathogens in the body, and scientology is a religion.

7. a. The hypothalamus-pituitary controls all endocrine glands. The thyroid gland is responsible for secreting T4 and T3, the pancreas secrets insulin, and the adrenal gland secretes mineralocorticoids and glucocorticoids.

8. d. The nervous system controls both voluntary and involuntary actions.

9. d. The study of the functions of the body is physiology. Kinesiology is the study of body movement, reflexology is the study of the feet and their nerves, and scientology is a religion.

10. a. The thyroid, which secretes T4 and T3, controls metabolism. The thymus is involved in immune function, the adrenal gland is responsible for secreting epinephrine, and the pituitary gland releases stimulating hormones.

11. d. The cardiac muscle is the only muscle that controls contractions of the heart. The smooth muscle pumps blood through vessels, the skeletal muscle causes movement, and the pericardium is a protective sac around the heart.

12. c. Arteries carry the oxygen-rich blood. Veins and vena cava carry oxygen-depleted blood, and atrium is not a vessel, it is a chamber.

13. d. The ovaries are the only organs listed that are in the pelvic cavity. The stomach and liver are found in the abdominal cavity, and the thyroid is in the thoracic cavity.

14. a. The generic name is also referred to as the common or general name. Brand, trade, and proprietary names are all the same thing.

15. a. The large intestine reabsorbs water to prevent dehydration. The small intestine is responsible for the absorption of nutrients, the stomach is responsible for the chemical breakdown, and the pancreas releases sodium bicarbonate.

16. b. The stomach breaks foods down chemically. The mouth is responsible for physical breakdown, the small intestine absorbs nutrients, and the large intestine is responsible for excretion.

17. a. The pancreas controls blood glucose levels by secreting insulin. The thyroid secretes T4 and T3, the pituitary secretes stimulating hormones, and the testes release sex hormones.

18. b. Diabetes is the condition where the body has a resistance or inability to produce insulin. Hypothyroidism occurs when there is a lack of thyroid hormone, polycystic ovarian syndrome occurs when there is an imbalance of sex hormones, and a growth disorder occurs when there is a lack or excess of growth hormone.

19. d. Pharmacokinetics is the study of how a drug moves and changes when in the body. The mechanism of action is how a medication works on the body, indication is the use of a medication, and pharmacodynamics is the study of the physiological changes that occur in the body.

20. b. Bronchitis is an inflammation of the bronchial tubes. Emphysema is the destruction of alveoli, URI is an infection, and cystic fibrosis is the production of thick, sticky mucus.

21. c. Absorption of nutrients and medications is the main function of the small intestines. The stomach is responsible for chemical breakdown, the large intestine is responsible for reabsorption of water, and the mouth is responsible for physical breakdown.

22. b. The adrenal gland secretes epinephrine, glucocorticoids, and mineralocorticoids. The thyroid gland secretes thyroid hormone, the pancreas secretes insulin, and the gonads release sex hormones.

23. b. The endocrine system does the communicating for the nervous system. The cardiovascular system pumps blood, the gastrointestinal digests food, and the musculoskeletal allows for movement.

24. d. Red marrow produces white blood cells, red blood cells, and platelets.

25. d. A stroke is a clot that travels to the brain blocking the flow of oxygen. CAD is the narrowing of coronary arteries, hypertension is high blood pressure, and a myocardial infarction is a heart attack.

26. a. A rash is an area of red, inflamed skin.

27. a. The study of the physiological effects a medication has on the body is called pharmacodynamics. Metabolism is how a medication is broken down, absorption is how a medication makes it into the body, and pharmacokinetics is the path the medication takes in the body.

28. b. Depression would be characterized by symptoms of sadness, irritability, and lack of concentration. Seizures are characterized by convulsions or involuntary muscle movements of the body, schizophrenia is characterized by abnormalities in a patient's perception or expression of reality; and anxiety would involve feelings of uneasiness, apprehension, fear, and worry.

29. c. The central nervous system contains the spinal cord. Motor structures, sensory receptors, and the autonomic nervous system are all part of the peripheral nervous system.

30. c. The adult human body contains 206 bones.

31. d. Hypertension is commonly known as high blood pressure.

32. a. A lack of dopamine causes the shaking that characterizes Parkinson's. Serotonin and monoamines are responsible for mood, while endorphins are a natural anesthetic.

33. b. If CAD is left untreated, it will cause a blockage of blood flow to the heart which will trigger a myocardial infarction. Migraines are triggered by a spasm in the vessels that supply blood to the brain, atrial flutter is caused by irregular electrical activity, and the AV node is part of the conduction system.

34. a. The top chambers of the heart are the atria. Ventricles are the bottom chambers.

35. c. Indication refers to a medication's use. Action is what the medication does, classification is the grouping of medications, and interaction is when a medication clashes with another.

36. b. A group of medications with similar characteristics is called a drug classification. Generics are a cost-effective medication, indication is the use, and action is what the medication does.

37. b. A loss of bone density is known as osteoporosis, which is commonly caused by menopause. Osteomyelitis is an infection, while arthritis and tendonitis are inflammatory conditions.

38. d. The human heart has four chambers: two atria and two ventricles.

39. c. An undesired effect from a medication is known as an adverse reaction. Indication is use, and action is how a medication works.

40. a. Pharmacokinetics is important in the dosing of medications that need to be exact as possible, such as in the hospital setting. This is a true statement.

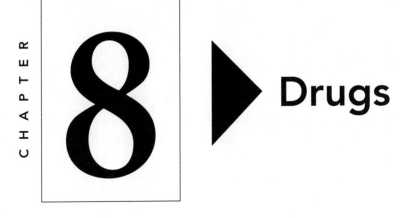

8 ▶ Drugs

CHAPTER OVERVIEW

The term *pharmacology* refers to how the drug works in the body, or what is called the mechanism of action, and how the drug works to treat specific disease states. As you have already reviewed some basic anatomy and physiology, this chapter will continue onward, using that information. This chapter will give you a basic understanding of what purpose a drug's classification serves in treating specific disease states. The main focus of this chapter is to simply learn the top 100 retail drugs in the pharmacy setting. With this in mind, you will be given a list of the top 100 retail drugs to memorize as much as possible. Since 20% of the exam does focus on this aspect, the more you know the better off you are going to be.

KEY TERMS

ACE inhibitors	benzodiazepines	drug class
adverse reactions	beta-blockers	fluoroquinolones
angiotensin 2 receptor antagonist	biguanide	generic name
anticonvulsant	cephalosporins	H1 blocker
antipsychotics	classification	H2 blocker
	cross-sensitivity	histamine 2 receptor antagonist

KEY TERMS (continued)

HMG-CoA reductase inhibitor	NSAID	sulfonamides
hypercholesterolemia	opiate agonists	sulfonylurea
main indication	penicillins	tetracyclines
MOA	proton pump inhibitor	trade name
non-benzodiazepines	SSRI	tricyclics

As a pharmacy technician, you will begin to build a basic understanding of drugs by learning about as many different drugs as you can. We will refer to the trade name, generic name, main indication, and classification of the drug. Most pharmacy technician programs require you to learn the top 200 drugs, but we will limit that to the top 100 drugs, which may seem overwhelming as well. Do not feel you need to know them all, but as mentioned before, the more you know the better prepared you will be when taking the national exam.

Drug Cards

To learn the four key pieces of information (**trade name**, **generic name**, **main indication**, and **classification**) about a specific drug, you will simply have to create your own method as far as memorization is concerned.

Cards with drug information written on them are useful, as they are easy to carry and do offer you the chance to test yourself. You can purchase 3 × 5 index cards to make your own drug cards. Preparing your own drug cards begins your learning process.

Information needed on your drug card:

- trade name of drug
- generic name of drug
- main indication
- classification
- any other useful information you may want to include

A sample drug card:

Esomeprazole

Nexium *GERD* **Proton Pump Inhibitor**

Side one: List the generic name.

Side two: Include the trade name, main indication, and classification.

Top 100 Drug List

The following table lists the top 100 retail drugs for you to memorize:

RANK	GENERIC NAME	SOME TRADE NAMES	MAIN INDICATION	CLASSIFICATION
1	hydrocodone/acetaminophen	Vicodin®, Lorcet®	pain	opiate agonist
2	levothyroxine	Synthroid®, Levothroid®	hypothyroidism	hormone (thyroid)
3	metoprolol	Lopressor®, Toprol®	hypertension	beta 1 blocker
4	lisinopril	Prinivil®, Zestril®	hypertension	ACE inhibitor
5	atorvastatin	Lipitor®	hypercholesterolemia	HMG-CoA reductase inhibitor
6	amoxicillin	Amoxil®, Trimox®	infection	penicillin
7	hydrochlorothiazide (HCTZ)	Microzide®, Esidrix®	hypertension	thiazide diuretic
8	azithromycin	Zithromax®	infection	macrolide
9	metformin	Glucophage®	type 2 diabetes	biguanide
10	atenolol	Tenormin®	hypertension	beta 1 blocker
11	simvastatin	Zocor®	hypercholesterolemia	HMG-CoA reductase inhibitor
12	alprazolam	Xanax®	anxiety	benzodiazepine
13	furosemide	Lasix®	hypertension	loop diuretic
14	zolpidem	Ambien®	isomnia	non-benzodiazepine
15	potassium chloride	K-Dur®, Klor-Con®, Micro-K®	hypokalemia	potassium electrolyte
16	sertraline	Zoloft®	depression	SSRI
17	montelukast	Singulair®	antihistamine	leukotriene inhibitor
18	escitalopram	Lexapro®	depression	SSRI
19	oxycodone/acetaminophen	Percocet®, Tylox®	pain	opiate agonist
20	esomeprazole	Nexium®	GERD	proton pump inhibitor
21	warfarin	Coumadin®	blood clots	anticoagulant
22	ibuprofen	Motrin®, Advil®	inflammation	NSAID
23	clopidogrel	Plavix®	clot prevention	platelet inhibitor
24	a mlodipine	Norvasc®	hypertension	calcium channel blocker
25	prednisone	Deltasone®	inflammation (adrenal) insufficiency	corticosteroid

RANK	GENERIC NAME	SOME TRADE NAMES	MAIN INDICATION	CLASSIFICATION
26	cephalexin	Keflex®	infection	cephalosporin
27	fluoxetine	Prozac®, Serafem®	depression	SSRI
28	albuterol	Ventolin®, Proventil®	bronchospasm	beta 2 agonist
29	ceftirizine	Zyrtec®	allergies	H1 blocker
30	triamterene/HCTZ	Dyazide®, Maxzide®	hypertension	diuretic combination
31	propoxyphene/ acetaminophen	Darvocet®, Wygesic®	pain	non-opiate agonist
32	lorazepam	Ativan®	anxiety	benzodiazepine
33	omeprazole	Prilosec®	GERD	proton pump inhibitor
34	lansoprazole	Prevacid®	GERD	proton pump inhibitor
35	clonazepam	Klonopin®	anxiety	benzodiazepine
36	tramadol	Ultram®	pain	non-opiate agonist
37	amoxicillin/clavulanate	Augmentin®	infection	penicillin
38	ezetimibe/simvastatin	Vytorin®	hypercholesterolemia	cholesterol absorption inhibitor/HMG-CoA reductase inhibitor
39	ciprofloxacin	Cipro®	infection	quinolone
40	cyclobenzaprine	Flexeril®	muscle spasm	skeletal muscle relaxant
41	fluticasone/Salmeterol	Advair Diskus®	asthma	steroid/bronchodilator
42	gabapentin	Neurontin®	seizures	anticonvulsant
43	sulfamethoxazole/ trimethoprim	Bactrim®, Septra®	infection	sulfonalamide
44	fexofenadine	Allegra®	allergies	H1 blocker
45	norgestimate	Ortho Tri-Cyclen®	birth control	birth control
46	venlafaxine	Effexor®	depression	antidepressant
47	lisinopril/hydro-chlorothiazide (HCTZ)	Zestorectic®, Prinzide®	hypertension	ACE inhibitor/thiazide diuretic
48	citalpram	Celexa®	depression	SSRI
49	pantoprazole	Prontonix®	GERD	proton pump inhibitor
50	paroxetine	Paxil®	depression	SSRI
51	trazodone	Desyrel®	depression	tricyclic
52	naproxen	Aleve®, Naprosyn®, Anaprox®	inflammation	NSAID
53	lovastatin	Mevacor®	hypercholesterolemia	HMG-CoA reductase inhibitor

RANK	GENERIC NAME	SOME TRADE NAMES	MAIN INDICATION	CLASSIFICATION
54	glipizide	Glucotrol®	type 2 diabetes	sulfonylurea
55	valsartan	Diovan®	hypertension	angiotensin 2 receptor blocker (A2RB)
56	alendronate	Fosamax®	osteoporosis	bone resorption inhibitor
57	fluticasone	Flovent®, Flonase Inhaler®	asthma	corticosteroid
58	ethinyl estradiol/ drospirenone	Yasmin®, Yaz®	birth control	birth control
59	ezetimibe	Zetia®	hypercholesterolemia	cholesterol absorption inhibitor
60	acetaminophen/ codeine	Tylenol® No. 2 Tylenol® No. 3 Tylenol® No. 4	pain	non-narcotic/opiate agonist
61	rosuvastatin	Crestor®	hypercholesterolemia	MHG-CoA reductase inhibitor
62	levofloxacin	Levaquin®	infection	quinolone
63	amitriptyline	Elavil®	depression	tricyclic
64	diazepam	Valium®	anxiety	benzodiazepine
65	enalapril	Vasotec®	hypertension	ACE inhibitor
66	valsartan/HCTZ	Diovan®	hypertension	A2RB
67	digoxin	Lanoxin®	tachycardia	inotrope
68	ranitidine	Zantac®	GERD	H2 blocker
69	duloxetine	Cymbalta®	depression	SSRI
70	fluconazole	Diflucan®	candidiasis	antifungal
71	pioglitazone	Actos®	type 2 diabetes	thiazolidinedione
72	bupropion	Wellbutrin®	depression	aminoketone
73	oxycodone	OxyContin®	pain	opiate agonist
74	carisoprodol	Soma®	muscle spasm	skeletal muscle relaxant
75	conjugated estrogen	Premarin®	menopause	hormone (estrogen)
76	allopurinol	Zyloprim®	gout	xanthine oxidase inhibitor
77	doxycycline	Vibramycin®, Doryx®	infection	tetracycline
78	diltiazem	Cardizem®, Dilacor®	hypertension	calcium channel blocker
79	methylprednisolone	Medrol®	inflammation	corticosteroid

RANK	GENERIC NAME	SOME TRADE NAMES	MAIN INDICATION	CLASSIFICATION
80	celecoxib	Celebrex®	pain, inflammation	COX-2 inhibitor
81	tamsulosin	Flomax®	prostate enlargement	prostate receptor antagonist
82	quetiapine	Seroquel®	schizophrenia	antipsychotic
83	clonidine	Catapres®	hypertension	alpha receptor agonist
84	mometasone	Nasonex®	allergies	corticosteroid
85	fenofibrate	Tricor®	hypercholesterolemia	lipid lowering agent
86	insulin glargine	Lantus®	type 1 or 2 diabetes	insulin
87	sildenafil	Viagra®	erectile dysfunction	5A-phosphodiesterase inhibitor
88	olanzapine	Zyprexia®	schizophrenia	antipsychotic
89	ramipril	Altace®	hypertension	ACE inhibitor
90	promethazine	Phenergan®	nausea	antiemetic
91	carvedilol	Coreg®	hypertension	beta 1 and 2 blocker
92	isosorbide mononitrate	Imdur®, Ismo®, Monoket®	angina	vasodilator
93	clindamycin	Cleocin®	infection	antibiotic
94	pravastatin	Pravachol®	hypercholesterolemia	HMG-CoA reductase inhibitor
95	amphetamine/ destroamphetamine	Adderall®	ADHD	CNS stimulant/ amphetamine
96	meloxicam	Mobic®	anti-inflammatory	NSAID
97	a mlodipine/ benazepril	Lotrel®	hypertension	calcium channel blocker/ACE inhibitor
98	risedronate	Actonel®	osteoporosis	bone resorption inhibitor
99	verapamil	Calan®, Covera®, Verelan®	hypertension	calcium channel blocker
100	cefdinir	Omnicef®	infection	cephalosporin

Trade Name versus Generic Name

When a drug manufacturer decides to produce a new drug for marketing, it will give the drug a trade name (also known as a brand name) and a generic name. Manufacturers hold a patent right (exclusive rights of ownership) for their new drug for 20 years. The trade name is the name the manufacturer uses to identify its product; it also helps identify that drug as being made by that specific drug manufacturer for marketing purposes. The generic name is what is known as the general or common name of the drug. This will be the name that follows that drug, even if the original manufacturer no longer produces that drug or if different companies produce it after the original company's patent right of 20 years has expired.

For example, the drug manufacturer Pfizer introduced Lipitor®, used as **hypercholesterolemia** (cholesterol-lowering) medication. Pfizer has exclusive rights to the name Lipitor® and its chemical composition for a certain period of time. Once that time has elapsed, other manufacturers may reproduce Lipitor® as its generic equivalent, atorvastatin, but may not use the trade name Lipitor®. Another example is Purdue Pharma's OxyContin®. Although Purdue retains the right to the name OxyContin®, other manufacturers produce its generic equivalent, oxycodone.

An interesting fact about why generic drugs are less expensive than the original trade name drugs is that generic drug companies simply do not have to do the drug development phase. This is when clinical studies and trials are done to prove the drug is safe and effective. Generic companies need only manufacture the drugs without drug development costs associated.

Main Indication

A drug's main indication describes what the drug is being used for—or, more specifically, which medical condition the drug treats. The terms *antidepressant* (for depression), *antihistamine* (for allergies), or *antihypertensive* (for high blood pressure) would be considered a main indication. The following table lists examples of some main indications:

MAIN INDICATION	WHAT THE DRUG IS USED FOR	EXAMPLE DRUG
analgesics	for chronic or acute pain	hydrocodone/acetaminophen (Vicodin®)
antacids	for heartburn or acid reflux	MgOH and AlOH (Maalox®)
antianginals	for chest pain associated with need for oxygen	nitroglycerin (Nitrostat®)
anticoagulents	to prevent blood clot formation	warfarin (Coumadin®)
anticonvulsants	for seizure control	carbamazepine (Tegretol®)
antidepressant	for depression	sertraline (Zoloft®)
antihistamines	for allergies	ceftirizine (Zyrtec®)
antihypertensives	to lower blood pressure	atenolol (Tenormin®)
antibiotics	for bacterial infection	amoxicillin (Amoxil®)
antineoplastics	for treatment of specific cancers	doxyrubicin (Adriamycin®)
anti-inflammatory agents	reduces inflammation	ibuprofen (Motrin®)

MAIN INDICATION	WHAT THE DRUG IS USED FOR	EXAMPLE DRUG
antitussives	for cough	dextromethorphan lozenges
antivirals	for viral infections	acyclovir (Zovirax®)
bronchodilators	for asthma	albuterol (Ventolin®)
digestants	to promote digestion of food	simethicone (Mylicon®)
diuretics	to increase urine output	HCTZ (Esidrex®)
hormones	to replace natural endogenous organic compounds	conjugated estrogens Premarin®)
hypnotics and sedatives	to inoduce and maintain sleep	zolpidem (Ambien®)
tranquilizers	reduces anxiety	lorazepam (Ativan®)

Classification of a Drug

The **classification** of a drug gives us information about a specific drug as to its chemical structure, **MOA** (or how the drug works in the body), and associated side or adverse effects. In knowing the **drug class**, we are given a more detailed explanation of how the drug works in the body when prescribing a drug for specific disease states. An example would be the antidepressant Prozac®, which treats depression. But there are other antidepressants as well, and they each treat depression in a different way. That is why we need to be more specific—not only knowing the category of the drug (antidepressant), but also the classification of the drug, which in the case of Prozac® is **serotonin-specific reuptake inhibitor (SSRI)**.

A classification of drug can be a subset of its main indication in that it is being used for a specific disease state, but its mechanism of action or how it works to treat that disease state may be different. An example would be the main indication antihypertensive, which is indicative of drugs used to treat high blood pressure. But there are different ways to treat this disease state, so we have different classifications of drugs that are a subset of the main indication.

Classifications of drugs to treat, for example, a high blood pressure disease state:

- ACE inhibitors
- alpha-2 agonists
- angiotensin 2 receptor blockers
- beta-adrenergic blockers
- calcium channel blockers
- cardiac glycosides
- diuretics

Classifications of drugs have three similarities which make them unique in treating a disease state. They all have a similar chemical structure, mechanism of action, and side (or adverse) effects. If you know the classification of a drug, you already know much about that specific drug. You do not need a pharmacist's clinical understanding of the classification of drugs. They are trained to be drug experts and understand the classification of drugs in an educational and scientific way. But that does not mean you should not have a basic understanding, as this will help you in the pharmacy setting you work in—especially if you get into the hospital/clinical aspect of pharmacy.

The following are a few examples to give you a better understanding of what classifications mean.

These classifications will also include drugs that are part of the list of top 100 retail drugs. The national exam may have one or two questions regarding the following information. In any case, the more you know, the better asset you will be as a pharmacy technician, and the more you will grow personally and professionally.

Antibiotics

Antibiotics are medications that have the ability to destroy or inhibit the development of living organisms, typically bacteria. Many of them are derived from the defense mechanisms used by other organisms, such as mold, to fight infection. In most cases, a patient's own immune system can overcome simple infections, eliminating the need for an antibiotic. The following is a list of some classifications of antibiotics.

Penicillins

Penicillins are natural (or semisynthetic) antibiotics that are produced from a certain species of fungus called *penicillium*. These are the most widely used bactericidal agents, but their cousin **cephalosporins** have also had an increase in use in the past ten years. Penicillins can be used as both a broad spectrum antibiotic and a narrow spectrum antibiotic. This means that some penicillins have the ability to treat multiple types of bacteria, while others treat a limited number of them. In addition, hypersensitivity (allergic reaction) will occur in nearly 10% of all patients who take these medications. Because of this, it is important for a technician to verify any allergies a patient may have prior to beginning antibiotic therapy. Should a patient have a true allergy to penicillin, the protocol is to give them a macrolide antibiotic, which would include the drug erythromycin or azithromycin (such as the Z-Pak®).

Indication

Penicillins are used for the treatment of a broad spectrum of bacterial microorganisms (e.g., streptococcal, pneumococcal, and gonococcal infections). In addition, they can be used as a prophylactic prior to surgery. The most common use as a prophylactic is during oral surgery or dental work.

Mechanism of Action

Penicillins work to eliminate bacteria by inhibiting the bacterial cell wall growth. As the penicillin prevents the cell wall from growing, the cell will rupture, causing death; this is known as cytolysis.

Common Adverse Reactions

The most common **adverse reactions** associated with penicillins include nausea, vomiting, diarrhea, and anaphylactic shock.

Example Drugs from the Top 100 List:

GENERIC NAME	COMMON TRADE OR BRAND NAME(S)
amoxicillin	Amoxil®, Trimox®
amoxicillin/clavulanate	Augmentin®

Cephalosporins

Cephalosporins are semisynthetic antibiotics that are pharmacologically and structurally related to penicillin. They are resistant to ß-lactamase, which provides them with an advantage over penicillins. Cephalosporins are broken down into four "generations," which identify a broader use of the medication for bacterial infections. They are used as a substitute for penicillins in patients who have resistant bacterial infections. It should also be noted that because of their relation to penicillins, there is a 5% chance that a patient who is allergic to penicillins is also allergic to cephalosporins. This is called **cross-sensitivity**.

Indication

Cephalosporins are used for the treatment of a broad spectrum of bacterial microorganisms (e.g., streptococcal, pneumococcal, and gonococcal infections). In addition, they can be used for oral surgery, neurosurgery, female reproductive system surgeries or procedures, orthopedic surgery, and heart procedures.

Mechanism of Action

Cephalosporins work to eliminate bacteria by inhibiting cell wall growth. As the cephalosporin prevents the cell wall from growing, the cell will rupture, resulting in cytolysis.

Common Adverse Reactions

The most common adverse reactions associated with cephalosporins include nausea, vomiting, diarrhea, and anaphylactic shock.

Example Drugs from the Top 100 List:

GENERIC NAME	COMMON TRADE OR BRAND NAME(S)
cefdinir	Omnicef®
cephalexin	Keflex®

Fluoroquinolones

Fluoroquinolones are synthetic antibiotics that are used to treat a broad spectrum of bacterial infections (gram-negative and gram-positive bacteria). They are more potent than the penicillins and are less likely to cause anaphylaxis. They are used in a wide variety of treatments, making them an easy choice for practitioners. Because of their effectiveness and ability to treat a broad spectrum of bacteria, a tolerance toward these medications is beginning to develop within the population.

Indication

Fluoroquinolones are used for the treatment of a broad spectrum of bacterial microorganisms. Specifically, they are used for urinary tract, upper respiratory tract, ophthalmic, and bone infections.

Mechanism of Action

Fluoroquinolones work to eliminate bacteria by damaging the bacterial DNA. Without functioning DNA, the bacteria cannot perform the functions necessary to sustain life (such as respiration, protein synthesis, and replication) and will die.

Common Adverse Reactions

The most common adverse reactions associated with fluoroquinolones include nausea, vomiting, dizziness, and an unpleasant taste.

Example Drugs from the Top 100 List:

GENERIC NAME	COMMON TRADE OR BRAND NAME(S)
ciprofloxacin	Cipro®
levofloxacin	Levaquin®

Sulfonamides

Sulfonamides are synthetic derivatives of sulfanilamide, which was the first medication to be proven effective for the prevention and cure of bacterial infection. These antibiotics are typically classified into three categories: short-acting, intermediate-acting, and long-acting. These classifications are made based on the amount of time it takes for these medications to be absorbed and excreted. When you hear that a patient is allergic to sulfa drugs, they are referring to this classification of drug.

Indication

Sulfonamides are commonly used to treat urinary tract infections, *E. coli*, and upper respiratory infections.

Mechanism of Action

Sulfonamides work to eliminate bacteria by inhibiting bacterial inflammatory and immune response. In living organisms, the response to injury is inflammation. If this is inhibited, it leaves the bacteria susceptible to further damage. Without these responses, the bacteria cannot fight the immune system and will die off.

Common Adverse Reactions

The most common adverse reactions associated with sulfonamides include anemia, thrombocytopenia (or low platelet levels), and hypersensitivity reactions.

Example Drugs from the Top 100 List:

GENERIC NAME	COMMON TRADE OR BRAND NAME(S)
sulfamethoxazole/ trimethoprim	Bactrim®, Septra®

Tetracyclines

Tetracyclines are semisynthetic antibiotics obtained from the cultures of a bacteria known as streptomyces. They are considered broad spectrum and maintain stability in acidic solutions, making these a strong choice for oral administration. The absorption of these antibiotics is impaired by the stomach contents. The most common impediment to absorption into the blood is milk and antacids.

Indication

Tetracyclines are commonly used to treat gram-negative and gram-positive bacteria, including rickettsia and chlamydia.

Mechanism of Action

Tetracyclines work to eliminate bacteria by inhibiting bacterial protein synthesis. Protein carries out specific duties necessary to sustain cell life. Without the ability to make protein, the bacteria will die off.

Common Adverse Reactions

The most common adverse reactions associated with tetracyclines include nausea, vomiting, diarrhea, rash, and anaphylactic shock.

Example Drugs from the Top 100 List:

GENERIC NAME	COMMON TRADE OR BRAND NAME(S)
doxycycline	Vibramycin®, Doryx®

Antihistamines

Antihistamines are medications that are used to treat the symptoms of allergies. Histamine, which is a chemical substance in the body, protects the body from environmental factors we become exposed to, such as pollen. It will initiate the allergic and inflammatory reaction one would experience during a reaction, helping to protect the body from damage. One classification of antihistamines is **histamine 1 (H1) blockers.**

Indication

H1 blockers are used for allergic reactions caused by histamine.

Mechanism of Action

H1 blockers block the effects of histamine at H1 receptor sites, which are found throughout the body and initiate an allergic reaction. This prevents the symptoms of an allergic reaction from occurring.

Common Adverse Reactions

The most common adverse reactions associated with H1 blockers include drowsiness, dizziness, headaches, and photosensitivity.

Example Drugs from the Top 100 List:

GENERIC NAME	COMMON TRADE OR BRAND NAME(S)
ceftirizine	Zyrtec®

Anti-Inflammatory Drugs

Anti-inflammatory agents are medications that treat allergies and respiratory diseases. They do so by reducing inflammation in the affected area. These include steroidal products. We always think of NSAID drugs as prescription medications, but there are over-the-counter anti-inflammatory drugs such as ibuprofen available as well. Following is a list of one classification of anti-inflammatory drugs:

Non-Steroidal Anti-Inflammatory Drugs

Indication

NSAIDs are used to treat allergies and respiratory conditions.

Mechanism of Action

NSAIDs reduce swelling and inflammation caused by irritants or injury.

Common Adverse Reactions

The most common adverse reactions associated with anti-inflammatory drugs include dryness, headache, nausea, dizziness, and cough.

Example Drugs from the Top 100 List:

GENERIC NAME	COMMON TRADE OR BRAND NAME(S)
ibuprofen	Motrin®, Advil®
meloxicam	Mobic®
naproxen	Aleve®, Naprosyn®, Anaprox®

Hypnotic Drugs

Hypnotic medications depress the central nervous system to reduce the desire for physical activity or to produce a calming effect. They are commonly used to induce sedation. **Non-benzodiazepines** are a classification of hypnotic medications.

Non-Benzodiazepines

Indication

Non-benzodiazepines are used to induce or maintain sleep or decrease anxiety.

Mechanism of Action

Non-benzodiazepines act on the GABA neurotransmitter to produce a calming effect.

Common Adverse Reactions

The most common adverse reactions associated with non-benzodiazepines include dizziness, drowsiness, loss of cognition, depression, and sleepwalking.

Example Drugs from the Top 100 List:

GENERIC NAME	COMMON TRADE OR BRAND NAME(S)
zolpidem	Ambien®

Behavior Disorder Drugs

Behavior disorder medications are used to treat a variety of mental illness. They are used as both an acute and chronic treatment of mental conditions, including psychosis or depression. **Antipsychotics** and **benzodiazepines** are classifications of behavior disorder medications.

Antipsychotics

Indication

Antipsychotics are used to control symptoms of psychosis and mood disorders.

Mechanism of Action

Antipsychotic medications work on specific neurotransmitters, such as dopamine and serotonin.

Common Adverse Reactions

The most common adverse reactions associated with antipsychotics include dizziness, drowsiness, loss of cognition, depression, and extrapyramidal side effects (EPS), which are associated with involuntary muscle movements throughout the body.

Example Drugs from the Top 100 List:

GENERIC NAME	COMMON TRADE OR BRAND NAME(S)
olanzapine	Zyprexia®
quetiapine	Seroquel®

Benzodiazepines

Benzodiazepines are medications that are used to treat anxiety disorders. In addition, they are used in both acute and chronic situations. They are becoming more common due to their safety, compared to older medications used to treat the same conditions.

Indication

Benzodiazepines are used to treat anxiety and sleep disorders.

Mechanism of Action

Benzodiazepines act by potentiating the effect of the GABA neurotransmitter, which produces a calming effect.

Common Adverse Reactions

The most common adverse reactions associated with benzodiazepines include dizziness, drowsiness, confusion, and depression.

Example Drugs from the Top 100 List:

GENERIC NAME	COMMON TRADE OR BRAND NAME(S)
alprazolam	Xanax®
clonazepam	Klonopin®
diazepam	Valium®
lorazepam	Ativan®

Tricyclic Antidepressants

Tricyclic antidepressants are medications that are used to treat depressive disorders. The therapeutic effectiveness is usually around 70%. They work by inhibiting the uptake of neurotransmitters that are responsible for affecting mood.

Indication

Tricyclic antidepressants are used to treat unipolar depression and regulation of sleep patterns.

Mechanism of Action

Tricyclic antidepressants inhibit the uptake of serotonin and norepinephrine.

Common Adverse Reactions

The most common adverse reactions associated with tricyclic antidepressants include confusion, sedation, and blurred vision.

Example Drugs from the Top 100 List:

GENERIC NAME	COMMON TRADE OR BRAND NAME(S)
amitriptyline	Elavil®
trazodone	Desyrel®

Selective Serotonin Reuptake Inhibitors

SSRIs are the most commonly prescribed class of antidepressants. They are also considered to have the fewest and least serious side effects as compared to other antidepressants.

Indication

SSRIs are used to treat major depressive disorders.

Mechanism of Action

SSRIs block the reuptake of serotonin into the neuron. This allows the neurotransmitter to stimulate the receptor site, producing the desired response.

Common Adverse Reactions

The most common adverse reactions associated with SSRIs include confusion, sedation, and blurred vision.

Example Drugs from the Top 100 List:

GENERIC NAME	COMMON TRADE OR BRAND NAME(S)
citalpram	Celexa®
escitalopram	Lexapro®
fluoxetine	Prozac, Serafem®
paroxetine	Paxil®

Anticonvulsants

Anticonvulsants are medications that are used to prevent or stop seizures. Seizures are caused by an excessive discharge of neuronal activity. The goal of this treatment is to regulate the discharge activity to a normal level. The targeted effect occurs a few weeks after the initial administration. There is no specific classification name for anticonvulsants.

Indication
Anticonvulsants are used to stop or prevent seizures.

Mechanism of Action
Anticonvulsants are believed to work by influencing the GABA neurotransmitters, which suppress the central nervous system.

Common Adverse Reactions
The most common adverse reactions associated with anticonvulsants include nausea, vomiting, diarrhea, tremor, and dizziness.

Example Drugs from the Top 100 List:

GENERIC NAME	COMMON TRADE OR BRAND NAME(S)
gabapentin	Neurontin®

Narcotic Analgesics

Narcotic analgesics, also known as opioids or **opiate agonists**, are medications that are used to treat more severe pain in patients. They can be either semisynthetic or derived naturally from the poppy plant. This class of medications also has a high risk for abuse.

Indication
Narcotic analgesics are used to treat moderate to severe pain.

Mechanism of Action
Narcotic analgesics alter the perception of and response to painful stimuli by stimulating the opiate receptors in the brain.

Common Adverse Reactions
The most common adverse reactions associated with narcotic analgesics include nausea, mental clouding, sedation, euphoria, withdrawal, and constipation.

Example Drugs from the Top 100 List:

GENERIC NAME	COMMON TRADE OR BRAND NAME(S)
hydrocodone/ acetaminophen	Vicodin®, Lorcet®
oxycodone	OxyContin®
oxycodone/ acetaminophen	Percocet®, Tylox®

Antihypertensive Drugs

Antihypertensive drugs are used to treat high blood pressure. The mechanism of action varies with what classification of drug is being used. Below is a list of some classifications of antihypertensive drugs:

Beta-Blockers

Beta-blockers (sometimes written as β-blocker) are also known as beta-adrenergic receptor antagonists or blockers, and they are used to treat hypertension, especially in younger patients. In addition, they are the medication of choice for patients after a heart attack because of its mechanism of action.

Indication

Beta-blockers are used mainly for hypertension, but are also used for other cardiac disease states such as cardiac arrhythmias (irregular heartbeat) and myocardial infarction (heart attack).

Mechanism of Action

Beta-blockers occupy the B1 receptor site, which will increase vasodilation and decrease both heart rate and blood pressure.

Common Adverse Reactions

The most common adverse reactions associated with beta-blockers include dizziness, sexual dysfunction, and vertigo.

Example Drugs from the Top 100 List:

GENERIC NAME	COMMON TRADE OR BRAND NAME(S)
carvedilol	Coreg®
atenolol	Tenormin®
metoprolol	Lopressor®, Toprol®

Angiotensin Converting Enzyme Inhibitors

Angiotensin converting enzyme (ACE) inhibitors are a class of medications that are used to reduce blood pressure. They work by inhibiting angiotensin Converting Enzyme (ACE) from forming angiotensin 1 to angiotension 2, which is a naturally occurring vasoconstrictor.

Indication

ACE inhibitors are used to treat hypertension.

Mechanism of Action

ACE inhibitors work by inhibiting the conversion of angiotensin 1 into angiotensin 2, which causes vasoconstriction in the body.

Common Adverse Reactions

The most common adverse reactions associated with ACE inhibitors include headache, dizziness, weakness, and joint pain.

Example Drugs from the Top 100 List:

GENERIC NAME	COMMON TRADE OR BRAND NAME(S)
enalapril	Vasotec®
lisinopril	Prinivil®, Zestril®
ramipril	Altace®
lisinopril/HCTZ	Zestorectic®, Prinzide®

Angiotensin 2 Receptor Antagonists

Angiotensin 2 receptor antagonists are medications used to treat hypertension by interfering with the the substance A2. One of the benefits of these medications is that they can be given once a day, which increases patient compliance.

Indication

A2 receptor antagonists are used to treat hypertension.

Mechanism of Action

A2 receptor antagonists block the effects of the A2 enzyme at receptor sites, preventing vasoconstriction.

Common Adverse Reactions

These are the only antihypertensive drugs that have no specific side effects.

Example Drugs from the Top 100 List:

GENERIC NAME	COMMON TRADE OR BRAND NAME(S)
valsartan	Diovan®

Antihyperlipidemic Drugs

Antihyperlipidemics are medications used to reduce high cholesterol and reduce the risk of heart attacks. In most cases, these agents work by reducing low density lipoproteins (LDL) and increasing high density lipoproteins (HDL). **HMG-CoA reductase inhibitors** are one classification of an antihyperlipidemic drug.

HMG-CoA Reductase Inhibitors

Indication

HMG-CoA reductase inhibitors are used to lower blood cholesterol.

Mechanism of Action

HMG-CoA reductase inhibitors work by limiting the HMG-CoA reductase synthesis, which is necessary to produce LDL, or "bad cholesterol," in the body.

Common Adverse Reactions

The most common adverse reactions associated with antihyperlipidemics include abdominal pain, headache, nausea, constipation, and blurred vision.

Example Drugs from the Top 100 List:

GENERIC NAME	COMMON TRADE OR BRAND NAME(S)
simvastatin	Zocor®
atorvastatin	Lipitor®
lovastatin	Mevacor®
pravastatin	Pravachol®
rosuvastatin	Crestor®

Stomach Anti-Acidic Drugs

Stomach anti-acidic drugs work by decreasing the amount of acid produced in the stomach. These drugs help in many disease states, such as gastrointestinal esophageal reflux disease (GERD) or simply acid reflux disease. Following is a classification of a stomach anti-acid drug:

Histamine 2 Receptor Antagonists or Blockers

Histamine 2 receptor antagonists, or H2 blockers, are medications used to lower the amount of gastric acid produced in the parietal cells of the stomach. These medications are also used to heal gastric or duodenal ulcers.

Indication

H2 receptor antagonists are used to treat hypersecretory conditions which cause an excess of stomach acid.

Mechanism of Action

H2 receptor antagonists work by inhibiting the interaction of histamine at H2 receptor sites.

Common Adverse Reactions

The most common adverse reactions associated with H2 receptor antagonists include headache and rash.

Example Drugs from the Top 100 List:

GENERIC NAME	COMMON TRADE OR BRAND NAME(S)
ranitidine	Zantac®

Proton Pump Inhibitors

Proton pump inhibitors are medications used to lower the amount of gastric acid produced in the stomach. These medications are also used when working to heal gastric or duodenal ulcers caused by H. pylori.

Indication

Proton pump inhibitors are used to treat hypersecretory conditions which cause an excess of stomach acid.

Mechanism of Action

Proton pump inhibitors prevent the transport of hydrogen to the gastric system, which decreases the amount of stomach acid that can be produced.

Common Adverse Reactions

The most common adverse reactions associated with proton pump inhibitors include nausea, vomiting, fatigue, and dizziness.

Example Drugs from the Top 100 List:

GENERIC NAME	COMMON TRADE OR BRAND NAME(S)
esomeprazole	Nexium®
lansoprazole	Prevacid®
omeprazole	Prilosec®
pantoprazole	Prontonix®

Antidiabetic Drugs

Antidiabetic medications are used to lower blood sugar in type 2 diabetic patients who have what is called hyperglycemia, or high blood sugar. Diabetes is one of the most common diseases in the United States, and its treatment options are far ranging. **Sulfonylureas** and **biguanides** are classifications of antidiabetic drugs.

Sulfonylureas

Indication

Sulfonylureas are used to treat type 2 diabetes, or non-insulin-dependent diabetes.

Mechanism of Action

Sulfonylureas stimulate the production of insulin in the beta cells of the pancreas.

Common Adverse Reactions

The most common adverse reactions associated with sulfonylureas include vomiting, headache, blurred vision, sedation, and confusion.

Example Drugs from the Top 100 List:

GENERIC NAME	COMMON TRADE OR BRAND NAME(S)
glipizide	Glucotrol®

Biguanides

Indication

Biguanides are used to treat type 2 diabetes, or non-insulin-dependent diabetes.

Mechanism of Action

Biguanides reduce hepatic glucose output and increase uptake of glucose.

Common Adverse Reactions

The most common adverse reactions associated with biguanides include vomiting, headache, blurred vision, sedation, and confusion.

Example Drugs from the Top 100 List:

GENERIC NAME	COMMON TRADE OR BRAND NAME(S)
metformin	Glucophage®

Practice Questions

1. In the case of penicillins, there is a 5% chance that a patient who is allergic to penicillins is also allergic to cephalosporins. What is this called?
   a. adverse reaction
   b. side effect
   c. cross-sensitivity
   d. hypersensitivity reaction

2. Which of the following medications is an antihyperlipidemic?
   a. Lipitor®
   b. Zoloft®
   c. digoxin
   d. Plavix®

3. Which of the following medications is used to treat a bacterial infection?
   a. Diflucan®
   b. Norvasc®
   c. amoxicillin
   d. Ativan®

4. Which of the following medications is the generic version of Zestril®?
   a. enalapril
   b. alprazolam
   c. metoprolol
   d. lisinopril

5. If a patient has a true allergy to the drug penicillin, which medication would most likely be given to him or her?
   a. cephalexin monohydrate
   b. erythromycin
   c. tetracycline
   d. ciprofloxacin

6. Which of the following medications is the brand name for atenolol?
   a. Toprol-XL®
   b. Lipitor®
   c. Tenormin®
   d. Zocor®

7. Which of the following medications is a macrolide antibiotic?
   a. Levaquin®
   b. Zithromax®
   c. cephalexin
   d. Augmentin®

8. Which of the following medications is the generic for Lasix®?
   a. HCTZ
   b. dyazide
   c. furosemide
   d. Nexium®

9. What is the MOA of ACE inhibitors?
   a. They work by connecting A to C and then to E.
   b. They work by inhibiting bacterial cell wall synthesis.
   c. They work by preventing the attachment of A2 to receptor sites.
   d. They work by inhibiting the conversion of the A1 enzyme into the A2 enzyme.

10. Which of the following medications is a beta-blocker?
    a. Lexapro®
    b. Ambien®
    c. Zocor®
    d. Toprol-XL®

11. Which of the following medications is the generic name for Proventil®?
a. salmeterol
b. prednisone
c. albuterol
d. Synthroid®

12. Which of the following medications is the brand name for a mlodipine?
a. Norvasc®
b. Toprol-XL®
c. Singulair®
d. Flonase®

13. Which of the following medications is used in patients with thyroid hormone deficiency?
a. Singulair®
b. Synthroid®
c. Plavix®
d. Premarin®

14. Which of the following medications are used for patients with hyperglycemia?
a. Xanax®
b. metformin
c. predinsone
d. Celebrex®

15. Which of the following medications is an SSRI?
a. enalapril
b. Allegra®
c. Prevacid®
d. Zoloft®

16. What is the brand name for escitalopram?
a. Zoloft®
b. Synthroid®
c. Lexapro®
d. Restoril®

17. Which of the following medications is the trade name for hydrocodone/acetaminophen?
a. Tylenol® No. 3
b. Percocet®
c. Vicodin®
d. Darvocet-N®

18. Which of the following medications is a cephalosporin antibiotic?
a. Cephalexin®
b. Augmentin®
c. amoxicillin
d. Zithromax®

19. Which of the following medications are used for insomnia?
a. Xanax®
b. metformin
c. zolpidem
d. atenolol

20. Which of the following medications is a corticosteroid?
a. lorazepam
b. Lipitor®
c. Norvasc®
d. prednisone

21. Which of the following medications is the generic for Nexium®?
a. metformin
b. esomeprazole
c. ranitidine
d. naproxen

22. Which of the following medications is available OTC?
a. ibuprofen
b. Lexapro®
c. Dyazide®
d. Flonase®

23. Which of the following is an example of a chemotherapy drug?
   a. doxyrubicin
   b. atenolol
   c. lisinipril
   d. azithromycin

24. Which of the following medications is the brand name version of simvastatin?
   a. Singulair®
   b. cephalexin
   c. Zocor®
   d. Levaquin®

25. Which of the following medications is the trade name for montelukast?
   a. Diovan®
   b. Lotrel®
   c. Altace®
   d. Singulair®

26. Which of the following medications is a PPI (proton pump inhibitor)?
   a. Toprol-XL®
   b. Prevacid®
   c. HCTZ
   d. Lipitor®

27. Which of the following medications is a beta-blocker?
   a. tramadol
   b. metoprolol
   c. gabapentin
   d. trazodone

28. Which of the following medications is used for depression?
   a. Prozac®
   b. Flonase®
   c. Altace®
   d. naproxen

29. Which of the following medications is the brand name of lorazepam?
   a. Allegra®
   b. tramadol
   c. Ativan®
   d. Levoxyl®

30. Which of the following medications is the generic of Plavix®?
   a. clopidogrel
   b. zolpidem
   c. metformin
   d. clonazepam

31. Which of the following medications is a sulfonylurea?
   a. Nasonex®
   b. Percocet®
   c. glipizide
   d. Cozaar®

32. Which of the following medications is used to treat infection?
   a. Lotrel®
   b. Advair®
   c. Augmentin®
   d. enalapril

33. Which of the following medications is the brand name for fluticasone/salmeterol?
   a. Seroquel®
   b. Flonase®
   c. Levaquin®
   d. Advair®

34. Which of the following medications is the generic for Fosamax®?
   a. levothyroxine
   b. alendronate
   c. amitriptyline
   d. Levaquin®

35. Which of the following medications is NOT an SSRI?
    a. Zoloft®
    b. Prozac®
    c. Effexor XR®
    d. Celexa®

36. Which of the following medications is used to prevent blood clots?
    a. Coumadin®
    b. Paxil®
    c. trazodone
    d. Lotrel®

37. Which of the following medications is the brand name for paroxetine?
    a. Zyrtec®
    b. clonazepam
    c. Paxil®
    d. Protonix®

38. Which of the following medications is the generic name for Klonopin®?
    a. Premarin®
    b. diovan
    c. levoxyl
    d. clonazepam

39. Which of the following medications is an H1 antagonist?
    a. Naproxen®
    b. Zyrtec®
    c. Flonase®
    d. tramadol

40. Which of the following medications is used to treat GERD?
    a. Protonix®
    b. trazodone
    c. Lotrel®
    d. enalapril

Answers and Explanations

1. c. This is what we would call a cross-sensitivity.

2. a. Lipitor® is an antihyperlipidemic. Zoloft® is for depression, digoxin is for arrhythmias, and Plavix® is for strokes.

3. c. Amoxicillin treats bacterial infections. Diflucan® is for fungal infections, Norvasc® is for blood pressure, and Ativan® is for anxiety.

4. d. Lisinopril is the generic name for Zestril®. Alprazolam is generic Xanax®, metoprolol is generic Lopressor®, and enalapril is generic Vasotec®.

5. b. The protocol would be to give a drug within the classification of macrolides, such as erythromycin or azithromycin (including the Z-Pak®).

6. c. Atenolol is also known as Tenormin®. Toprol-XL® is known as metoprolol, Lipitor® is also known as atrovastatin, and Zocor® is known as simvastatin.

7. b. Zithromax® is a macrolide. Levaquin® is a quinolone, cephalexin is a cephalosporin, and Augmentin® is a penicillin.

8. c. Lasix is furosemide. HCTZ is hydrochlorothiazide, triamterene/HCTZ is Dyazide®, and esomperazole is Nexium®.

9. d. ACE inhibitors, or angiotensin-converting enzyme inhibitors, work by preventing the conversion of angiotensin 1 to angiotensin 2, which causes vasoconstriction and high blood pressure.

10. d. Toprol-XL® is the beta-blocker. Lexapro® is an SSRI, Zocor® is an antihyperlipidemic, and Ambien® is a hypnotic.

11. c. Albuterol is Proventil®. Salmeterol is Serevent®, prednisone is Pred Forte®, and Synthroid® is levothyroxine.

12. a. Norvasc® is a mlodipine. Singulair® is montelukast, Toprol-XL® is metoprolol, and Flonase® is fluticasone.

13. b. Synthroid®. Singulair® is for allergies, Plavix® is for strokes, and Premarin® is for menopause.

14. b. Metformin is used to treat hyperglycemia. Xanax® is used for anxiety, prednisone is for allergies and inflammation, and Celebrex® is for inflammation.

15. d. Zoloft® is an SSRI. Enalapril is an ACE inhibitor, Prevacid® is a proton pump inhibitor, and Allegra® is an antihistamine.

16. c. Lexapro® is escitalopram. Zoloft® is certraline, Synthroid® is levothyroxine, and Restoril® is temazepam.

17. c. Vicodin® is hydrocodone with acetaminophen, Tylenol® No. 3 is acetaminophen with 30 mg codeine, Percocet® is oxycodone with acetaminophen, and Darvocet-N® is propoxyphene napsylate.

18. a. Cephalexin® is a cephalosporin. Amoxicillin and Augmentin® are penicillin, and Zithromax® is macrolide.

19. c. Zolpidem is used for insomnia. Xanax® is for anxiety, metformin is for diabetes, and atenolol is for hypertension.

20. d. Prednisone is a corticosteroid. Lorazepam is a benzodiazepine, Norvasc® is a beta-blocker, and Lipitor® is an antihyperlipidemic.

21. b. Esomeprazole is the generic for Nexium®. Ranitidine is the generic for Zantac®, metformin is the generic for Glucophage®, and naproxen is the generic for Naprosyn®.

22. a. Ibuprofen is available over-the-counter with different trade names such as Motrin®.

23. a. Doxyrubicin, or Adriamycin®, would be an example of a chemotherapy drug used to treat cancer. Other examples of chemo drugs would be 5-fluorouracil (5FU) and Cisplatin®.

24. c. Zocor® is the brand name for simvastatin. Singulair® is the brand name for montelukast, Keflex® is the brand name for cephalexin, and Levaquin® is the brand name for levafloxicin.

25. d. Montelukast is the generic of Singulair®. Diovan®, Lotrel®, and Altace® are all brand names.

26. b. Prevacid® is a PPI. Toprol-XL® is a beta-blocker, HCTZ is a diuretic, and Lipitor® is an antihyperlipidemic.

27. b. Metoprolol is a beta-blocker. Tramadol is a synthetic opioid, gabapentin is an anticonvulsant, and trazodone is an antidepressant.

28. a. Prozac® is an antidepressant. Altace® is an ACE inhibitor, Flonase® a steroid, and naproxen is an NSAID.

29. c. Ativan® is the brand name for lorazepam. Allegra® is the brand name for fexofenadine, Ultram® is the brand name for tramadol, and Levoxyl® is the brand name for levothyroxine.

30. a. Clopidogrel is the generic version of Plavix®. Metformin is the generic name for Glucophage®, zolpidem is the generic name for Ambien®, and clonazepam is the generic name for Klonopin®.

31. c. Glipizide is a sulfonylurea, Percocet® is an opiate agonist, Nasonex® is a steroid, and Cozaar® is an A2 receptor antagonist.

32. c. Augmentin® is used to treat infection. Lotrel® is for high blood pressure, Advair® is for asthma, and enalapril is for blood pressure.

33. d. Advair is the brand name for fluticasone/salmeterol. Seroquel® is the brand name of quietapine, Levaquin® is the brand name of levafloxacin, and Flonase® is the brand name of fluticasone.

34. b. Alendronate is the generic name for Fosamax®. Levothyroxine is the generic name for Levoxyl®, amitriptyline is the generic name for Elavil®, and Levaquin® is the brand name of levafloxacin.

35. c. Effexor XR® is not an SSRI; the other drugs are SSRIs.

36. a. Coumadin® prevents blood clots. Trazodone and Paxil® treat depression. Lotrel® treats hypertension.

37. c. Paroxetine is the generic name for Paxil®.

38. d. Klonopin® is the brand for clonazepam. Premarin® is the brand name for conjugated estrogens, Levoxyl® is the brand name for levothyroxine, and Diovan® is the brand name for valsartan.

39. b. Zyrtec® is an H1 antagonist, or blocker. Naproxen® is an NSAID, Flonase® is a steroid, and tramadol is a synthetic opioid.

40. a. Protonix® is used to treat GERD. Lotrel® and enalapril treat hypertension, and trazodone treats depression.

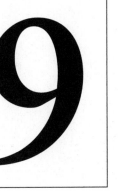

Pharmacy Math I

CHAPTER OVERVIEW

In some pharmacy settings, solving mathematical problems is necessary—especially in the hospital setting, where IV admixtures are made each day using calculations. The pharmacy technician exam will have a great many calculation problems; therefore, this chapter will focus specifically on the type of problem solving necessary for not only the national exam, but also the pharmacy setting you may choose to work in. A basic understanding of mathematics is necessary for the material covered in this and subsequent chapters involving calculations. This chapter will go over some basic mathematics as a review but will mainly focus on the problem solving you will see on the pharmacy technician exams. Specifically, this chapter will cover the concentration type of problem solving. To complete this chapter, you will need a basic calculator that adds, subtracts, divides, and multiplies. There is no need to get a pricey calculator or scientific calculator; when you take one of the national exams, you will be given a basic calculator to use.

KEY TERMS

Arabic numbers	metric system
common fraction	mixed fraction
complex fraction	numerator
concentration	proper fraction
decimal fraction	proportion
decimal number	ratio
denominator	Roman numerals
extremes	rounding
fraction	solute
improper fraction	solution
lowest common denominator	solvent
means	

There are three main types of problem solving done in the pharmacy: concentration, conversions, and percents. There are additional, secondary types of problem solving as well, such as pricing and temperature conversions. This chapter, as mentioned, will review (assuming you already have a basic understanding) mathematical skills as well as the first primary type of pharmacy problem solving, concentrations.

Fundamentals of Calculations

Calculations in the pharmacy setting require you have a basic understanding of **Roman numerals**, **Arabic numbers** we have used from childhood (1, 2, 3, 4, 5, 6, 7, 8, 9, 10, etc.), and critical thinking (the ability to look at a problem and figure out steps necessary to solve it).

Roman Numerals

In pharmacy practice, we may use Roman numerals to denote quantities ordered on prescriptions or when compounding, especially when using the apothecary system of weights and measures.

A numeral is a word or sign, or a group of words or signs, which express a number. The easiest way to note a number is to make that many marks—little I's. Thus I would mean 1, II would mean 2, and III would mean 3, and so on. However, this system becomes awkward and clumsy for larger numbers.

In the Roman system of counting, letters are used to designate numbers. Upper and lower case letters signify the same values (e.g., i = I). There are seven letters which represent Roman numerals: I, V, X, L, C, D, and M.

Arabic and Roman Numeral Equivalents

ARABIC NUMBER	ROMAN NUMERAL
½	ss
1	I or i*
2	II or ii
3	III or iii
4	IV or iv
5	V or v
6	VI or vi
7	VII or vii
8	VIII or viii
9	IX or ix

Arabic and Roman Numeral Equivalents

ARABIC NUMBER	ROMAN NUMERAL
10	X or x
20	XX or xx
30	XXX or xxx
40	XL or xl
50	L or l
100	C or c
500	D or d
1,000	M or m

* All lowercase Roman numerals may be written with a line above them.

In general, Roman numerals can be converted to Arabic numbers mathematically by simply assigning a numerical value to each letter and calculating a total. Although the historical practice has varied, the modern convention is to arrange the letters from left to right, in order of decreasing value; the total is then calculated by adding the numerical values of all the letters in the sequence. For example, the Roman numeral MDCLXXXVIII would be equal to:

$$1{,}000 + 500 + 100 + 50 + 10 + 10 + 10 + 5 + 1 + 1 + 1 = 1{,}688$$

Using this notation, Roman numerals can get quite long—and so the Romans began to use contractions, called the subtraction principle, in which a smaller letter appears before a larger letter to indicate a smaller number: IV = one from five = 4 or CM = one hundred from one thousand = 900.

There is one additional "Roman" numeral used in pharmacy practice, but was never used by the Romans: ss = $\frac{1}{2}$. You should be aware of this notation, but avoid its use. It is easily confused with the number 55 when handwritten and could lead to significant medication errors.

A simple set of rules governs the Roman system of notation in pharmacy practice. The position of one letter to another is very important and determines the value of the Roman numeral. Repeating a Roman numeral twice doubles its value; repeating a Roman numeral three times triples its value.

$$I = 1 \text{ and } II = 2$$

$$x = 10 \text{ and } xxx = 30$$

However, Roman numerals are not repeated more than three times in succession.

$$III = 3 \text{ is a correct notation, but } IIII = 4 \text{ is incorrect.}$$

When you place the same or a smaller Roman numeral after a larger Roman numeral, you add the Roman numerals together to calculate the Arabic (numeric) equivalent:

$$vi = v + i = 5 + 1 = 6$$

$$LX = L + X = 50 + 10 = 60$$

$$XXXI = X + X + X + I = 10 + 10 + 10 + 1 = 31$$

When you place a smaller Roman numeral before a larger Roman numeral, you subtract the smaller Roman numeral from the larger to calculate the Arabic equivalent:

$$IV = V - I = 5 - 1 = 4$$

$$ix = x - i = 10 - 1 = 9$$

$$XL = L - X = 50 - 10 = 40$$

When a Roman numeral of a smaller value comes between two of larger values, the subtraction rule is applied first, then the addition rule.

$$XIV = X + (V - I) = 10 + (5 - 1) = 10 + 4 = 14$$

$$XXIX = X + X + (X - I) = 10 + 10 + (10 - 1) = 10 + 10 + 9 = 29$$

$$xciv = (c - x) + (v - i) = (100 - 10) + (5 - 1) = 90 + 4 = 94$$

Numbers

A number is a total quantity or amount that is made up of one or more numerals. There are several kinds of numbers, including whole numbers; proper, improper, mixed, and **complex fractions**; and decimals. Examples of whole numbers include 10, 220, 5, and 19; examples of **fractions** include $\frac{1}{4}$, $\frac{2}{7}$, $\frac{4}{3}$, and $13\frac{3}{4}$; and examples of decimals include 3.6, 44.907, and 0.33.

Fractions

Fractions express a quantity that is a part or portion of a whole number or amount. A **common fraction** is an expression of division. The number below the fraction line is the **denominator**. The denominator indicates the total number of parts into which the whole is divided. The number above the fraction line is the **numerator**. The numerator indicates how many of those parts are considered.

Numerator (1 part)

Denominator (4 parts) $\qquad \frac{1}{4}$

A **proper fraction** has a numerator that is smaller than the denominator, and therefore always has a value of less than 1. For example, the common fraction three-quarters ($\frac{3}{4}$) is less than the whole (1).

Improper fractions have a numerator that is equal to or larger than the denominator, like the improper fraction three-halves ($\frac{3}{2}$). An improper fraction has a value greater than or equal to 1.

When the numerator and the denominator are equal, the value of the improper fraction is always 1, since a number divided by itself is always 1 ($\frac{4}{4} = 1$).

Unless directed otherwise or when carrying out a calculation, always express a fraction in its simplest form by reducing it to its lowest denominator. For **example:**

$$\frac{2}{4} = \frac{1}{2}$$

$$\frac{10}{12} = \frac{5}{6}$$

$$\frac{8}{12} = \frac{2}{3}$$

Mixed fractions contain both whole numbers and fractions. An improper fraction is reducible to either a whole number or a mixed fraction:

$$\frac{3}{2} = 1\frac{1}{2} \qquad \frac{8}{6} = \frac{4}{3} = 1\frac{1}{3} \qquad \frac{81}{27} = \frac{9}{3} = \frac{3}{1} = 3$$

Converting Mixed Fractions to Improper Fractions

It is important to be able to convert among different types of fractions. Conversion allows you to perform various calculations easier and permits you to express answers in simplest terms. To convert a mixed fraction to an improper fraction with the same denominator, multiply the whole number by the denominator and add the numerator. Then put this number over the original denominator.

Examples:

$$1\frac{5}{8} = \frac{(1 \times 8 + 5)}{8} = \frac{13}{8}$$

$$2\frac{3}{4} = \frac{(2 \times 4 + 3)}{4} = \frac{11}{4}$$

To convert an improper fraction to an equivalent mixed fraction or whole number, divide the numerator by the denominator. Express any remainder as a proper fraction and reduce to lowest terms.

Example: Express the improper fraction $\frac{8}{5}$ as a mixed fraction.

$$\frac{8}{5} = 8 \div 5 = 1\frac{3}{5}$$

Equivalent Fractions

You can express the value of a fraction in several ways. This is called *finding an equivalent fraction*. You either multiply or divide both terms of the fraction (numerator and denominator) by the same number to find an equivalent fraction. The form of the fraction is changed, but the value of the fraction remains the same.

When calculating dosages, it is usually easier to work with fractions of the smallest numbers possible. This concept of finding equivalent fractions is called *reducing the fraction to the lowest terms*, or simplifying the fraction. To reduce a fraction to lowest terms, divide the largest whole number that will go evenly into both the numerator and the denominator.

Example: Reduce $\frac{6}{12}$ to lowest terms.

Six is the largest number that will divide evenly into both 6 and 12:

$$\frac{6}{6} = 1 \text{ and } \frac{12}{6} = 2; \text{ therefore, } \frac{6}{12} = \frac{1}{2}$$

Note: If both numerator and denominator cannot be divided evenly by a whole number, the fraction is already in lowest terms.

To find an equivalent fraction in which both terms are larger than the original fraction, multiply both the numerator and the denominator by the same number.

Example: Enlarge $\frac{3}{5}$ to the equivalent fraction in tenths.

$$5 \times 2 = 10 \text{ and } 3 \times 2 = 6; \text{ therefore, } \frac{3}{5} = \frac{6}{10}$$

Lowest Common Denominator

The **lowest common denominator** (LCD) is the smallest whole number that can be divided evenly by all denominators. You must convert fractions to the LCD in order to add or subtract them. The first step in finding the LCD is to notice if one of the denominators is evenly divisible by the other denominators. If so, you have found the LCD.

Example: Find the lowest common denominator of $\frac{1}{5}$ and $\frac{4}{15}$. In this example, 15 is evenly divisible by 5, so 15 is the LCD.

Example: Find the lowest common denominator of $\frac{4}{9}$, $\frac{1}{3}$, and $\frac{1}{27}$. In this example, 27 is evenly divisible by 3 and 9, so 27 is the LCD.

Sometimes it is necessary convert a fraction into an equivalent fraction with the lowest common denominator you have found. The first step is to use the LCD to divide the denominator of the fraction to be changed. Then, multiply this number by the numerator of the fraction to be changed. Lastly, use the product as the numerator over the lowest common denominator.

Example:

$$\frac{5}{7} = \frac{x}{28}$$

$$28 \div 7 = 4$$

$$4 \times 5 = 20$$

Therefore,
$$\frac{5}{7} = \frac{20}{28}$$

Example:

$$\frac{3}{8} = \frac{x}{40}$$

$$40 \div 8 = 5$$

$$5 \times 3 = 15$$

Therefore,
$$\frac{3}{8} = \frac{15}{40}$$

You may also have to determine a fraction equivalent to a mixed number with the lowest common denominator. An improper fraction must first be determined from the mixed number. Then, divide the lowest common denominator by the denominator of the fraction and multiply this answer by the numerator of the improper fraction. Finally, use the product as the numerator over the lowest common denominator.

Example:

$$1\frac{3}{4} = \frac{x}{16}$$

Change $1\frac{3}{4}$ to an improper fraction…
$$\frac{4 \times 1 + 3}{3} = \frac{7}{4}$$

…which now makes the equation…
$$\frac{7}{4} = \frac{x}{16}$$

$$16 \div 4 = 4$$

$$4 \times 7 = 28$$

Therefore,
$$\frac{7}{4} = \frac{28}{16}$$

Or,
$$\frac{28}{16} = 1\frac{3}{4}$$

Finally, sometimes the lowest common denominator is not included in the denominators given in the problem. If this is the case, you must determine the LCD by trial and error. There are two approaches that can help in determining the LCD. One approach is to multiply the two given denominators together. If this makes a number that is too large to work with, another suggestion is to multiply the given denominators by 2, 3, or 4 to see if an LCD can be established.

Example:

Find the LCD for these two fractions:	$5\frac{1}{5}$ and $\frac{2}{3}$
Multiply the two denominators:	$5 \times 3 = 15$
	$5\frac{1}{5} = \frac{x}{15}$
	$\frac{5 \times 5 + 1}{5} = \frac{26}{5}$
So,	$\frac{26}{5} = \frac{x}{15}$
	$15 \div 5 = 3$
	$3 \times 26 = 78$
Thus,	$5\frac{1}{5} = \frac{78}{15}$

Decimals

The zero and the counting numbers (1, 2, 3, . . .) make up the set of whole numbers. But not every number is a whole number. Our decimal system lets us write numbers of all types and sizes, using a clever symbol called the decimal point, which looks like a period. As you move left from the decimal point, each place value is multiplied by 10, and as you move right from the decimal point, each place value is divided by 10.

Decimal numbers are another means of writing fractions, whole, and mixed numbers. You can identify decimal numbers by the period appearing within the number. The period in a decimal number is called the decimal point. Decimal numbers with a value less than one are **decimal fractions**; for example, 0.5, 0.003, and 0.75 are decimal fractions. Decimal fractions are fractions with a denominator of 10, 100, 1,000, or any multiple or power of 10. The position of the number in relation to the decimal point indicates its value.

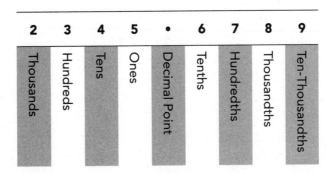

The number in the example above is 2,345.6789, which is read "two thousand, three hundred forty-five and six thousand seven hundred eighty-nine ten-thousandths."

Example: Look carefully at the decimal fraction 0.375. This is the same as three hundred seventy-five thousandths. You can see that 0.375 is less than 0.87 (eighty-seven hundredths), but greater than 0.0125 (one hundred twenty-five ten-thousandths).

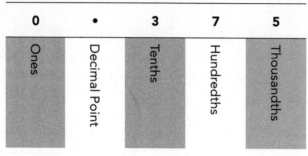

0	•	3	7	5
Ones	Decimal Point	Tenths	Hundredths	Thousandths

Zeros added after the last digit of a decimal fraction do not change its value: 0.375 = 0.3750. Zeros added between the decimal point and the first digit of a decimal fraction do change its value: 0.375 ≠ 0.0375.

To eliminate confusion, the following points about zeros are very important:

- Do not write a whole number in decimal form: 5 is correct; 5.0 is wrong.
- Do not write a decimal number with "trailing zeros": 5.2 is correct; 5.20 is wrong.
- When writing a fraction in decimal form, always precede the decimal point with a zero: 0.5 is correct;. 5 is wrong.

Rounding Decimal Numbers

For most pharmacy dosage calculations, it will only be necessary to carry decimals to thousandths (three decimal places) and **round** back to hundredths (two places) for the final answer. You may also need to round to tenths in some cases.

To round a decimal to hundredths, drop the number in the thousandths place and:

- Do not change the number in the hundredths place if the number in the thousandths place is 4 or less.
- Increase the number in the hundredths place by 1 if the number in the thousandths place is 5 or greater.

Example: Round the following decimals to two places (hundredths):

0.123 = 0.12

1.744 = 1.74

0.006 = 0.01

5.315 = 5.32

5.325 = 5.33

0.666 = 0.67

Fractions can also be changed into decimals by simply dividing the numerator (top number) by the denominator (bottom number).

Example: Write $\frac{3}{20}$ as a decimal.

Simply divide 3 by 20 to get your decimal number: 0.15.

Units of Measurement

In pharmacy calculations, the units of measure are mostly from the **metric system** for strengths of medications and volumes of medication. There are exceptions which will be covered later, but it is safe to say that most calculations problems you will find on the national exam and in the pharmacy setting involve the microgram (mcg), milligram (mg), gram (g), and kilogram (kg) as units of measure for weight and milliliter (ml or mL) and liter (L) as units of measure for volume.

Liquid volume is measured in liters or milliters.

> Liter is L
>
> Milliliter is ml
>
> 1L = 1,000 ml

The measure of weight is a little bit more involved.

LARGEST NUMBER			SMALLEST NUMBER
kilogram	gram	milligram	microgram
(kg)	(g)	(mg)	(mcg)
kilogram is **kg**	gram is **g**	milligram is **mg**	microgram is **mcg**

Ratio and Proportion

Since **ratio** and **proportion** can be used in solving 95% of problems you will find on the exam as well as in the pharmacy setting, we will use this methodology as the core of most calculations problem solving in this book. This type of problem solving is what is known as basic algebra, but no experience in algebra is necessary if you simply follow the steps needed to solve.

A ratio states the relative size relationship between two quantities expressed as the quotient of one divided by the other. For example, if there are 5 g of dextrose in 100 ml of sterile water, you express the ratio as $\frac{5}{100}$, or 5:100.

A ratio is a mathematical expression that indicates a relationship of one part of a quantity to the whole.

When written out, the two quantities are separated by a colon. For example, if you are considering five parts out of a total of nine parts, it can be expressed as the ratio 5:9 or as the fraction $\frac{5}{9}$. When you express this ratio verbally, you would say "five is to nine." *In problem solving, you will find most ratios will be stated as a fraction.*

A proportion expresses the relationship between two equal ratios. For example, a proportion may be expressed as two equal fractions:

$$\frac{5}{10} = \frac{15}{30}$$

This expression would be spoken as "5 is to 10 as 15 is to 30."

The two inside terms in a proportion are called the **means**. The two outside terms in a proportion are called the **extremes**.

In the example above, 5 and 30 are the extremes, and 10 and 15 are the means. In a proportion, the product of the means is equal to the product of the extremes. In the same example, $5 \times 30 = 10 \times 15 = 150$.

The usefulness of a proportion lies in the fact that if you know three of the four terms in a proportion, you can calculate the unknown fourth term. Proportion will be the single most useful tool that you will use for pharmaceutical calculations.

Example: $\frac{5}{10} = \frac{15}{30}$

x is the unknown number for which the equation is to be solved.

Solving Problems by the Ratio and Proportion Method

The ratio and proportion method is an accurate and simple way to solve some problems. In order to use this method, you should learn how to arrange the terms correctly, and you must know how to multiply and divide.

Term #1/Term #2 = Term #3/Term #4

"Term #1 is to Term #2 as Term #3 is to Term #4." Term #1 and Term #4 are the extremes and Term #2 and Term #3 are the means. By cross multiplying Term #1 with Term #4 and Term #2 with Term #3, the proportion can now be written as:

(Term #1) × (Term #4) = (Term #2) × (Term #3)

If you know any three of these terms, you can use this equation to solve for the unknown fourth term.

A good way to set up your proportion is to always write what information you have (your first ratio) equal to what information you want (your second ratio).

have = want

Example: How many grams of dextrose are in 10 ml of a solution containing 50 g dextrose in 100 ml of water?

Set up the proportion: have = want

50 g/100 ml = x g/10 ml

Cross multiply to get this equation: (parentheses indicate multiplication)

$$(x \text{ g}) (100 \text{ ml}) = (50 \text{ g}) (10 \text{ ml})$$

Solve for x by dividing both sides by 100 ml: $x \text{ g} = (50 \text{ g}) (10 \text{ ml})/(100 \text{ ml}) = 5 \text{ g}$

Let us look at this one again and see the steps one by one:

$$\frac{50 \text{ g}}{100 \text{ ml}} = \frac{x \text{ g}}{10 \text{ ml}}$$

$$\frac{\text{Extremes}}{\text{Means}} = \frac{\text{Means}}{\text{Extremes}}$$

$$(\text{Means}) (\text{Means}) = (\text{Extremes}) (\text{Extremes})$$

$$(x \text{ g}) (100 \text{ ml}) = (50 \text{ g}) (10 \text{ ml})$$

$$(x \text{ g}) = (50 \text{ g}) (10 \text{ ml})/(100 \text{ ml})$$

$$x \text{ g} = 5 \text{ g}$$

Concentration Problem Solving

A **concentration** is the amount of a **solute** (active drug) in a **solution** per standard amount of **solvent** (solution).

- solution: a mixture consisting of a solute and a solvent
- solute: component of a solution present in the lesser amount
- solvent: component of a solution present in a great amount

A more concentrated solution would have a great deal of solute per solvent (solution) present. A lesser concentration would be the opposite, where the solvent (solution) is much greater than the solute.

Example: 1 mg/100 ml is going to have a lesser concentration than 10 mg/100 ml and even less concentration than a 50 mg/100 ml solution.

In liquid medication preparations, there is a specific amount of drug per a specific volume in milliliters, which is known as a concentration. A concentration is defined in pharmacy as the amount of active drug in grams over a specific volume.

Example: 250 mg/5 ml

The example tells us there is 250 mg of active drug per 5 ml of solution. If this were the drug amoxicillin, it would be 250 mg of amoxicillin per 5 ml of solution. In oral liquid preparations, the concentration generally has a specific volume of 5 ml, as this is equal to one teaspoonful. This is not the case of IV admixtures, where concentrated injectable drugs will have different specific volumes in their concentration. An example of this would be the drug ampicillin (for injection), which may have a concentration of 250 mg active drug per 2 ml solution.

Example: If a concentration of drug is 400 mg/5 ml, how many milligrams will a 12 ml dose give?

have = want

Setup: 400 mg/5 ml = x mg/12 ml

If you see a concentration in your problem, this will be what you "have" in setting up your proportion!

Cross multiply to get this equation: (400 mg) (12 ml) = (x mg) (5 ml)

Solve for x by dividing both sides by 5 ml: (400 mg) (12 ml)/(5 ml) = 960 mg

Example: If a cough syrup contains 4 mg of chlorpheniramine in each 5 ml, how much chlorpheniramine in mg is contained in 240 ml of syrup?

Setup: 4 mg/5 ml = x mg/240 ml

Cross multiply to get this equation: (4 mg) (240 ml) = (x mg) (5 ml)

Solve for x by dividing both sides by 5 ml: (4 mg) (240 ml)/(5 ml) = 192 mg

Example: You need to prepare a 100 mg dose of amoxicillin. The concentration of the suspension (liquid formulation) is 250 mg/5 ml. How many milliliters will be needed to give a 100 mg dose?

Set up the proportion: 250 mg/5 ml = 100 mg/x ml

Cross multiply to get this equation: (250 mg) (x ml) = (100 mg) (5 ml)

Solve for x by dividing both sides by 250 mg: x ml = (100 mg)(5 ml)/(250 mg) = 2 ml

Example: Erythromycin ethylsuccinate (EES) comes in a liquid suspension with a concentration of 333 mg/5 ml. If you are asked to give an exact dose of 200 mg, how many milliliters are needed?

Set up the proportion: 333 mg/5 ml = 200 mg/x ml

Cross multiply to get this equation: (333 mg) (x ml) = (200 mg) (5 ml)

Solve for x by dividing both sides by 333 mg: x ml = (200 mg)(5 ml)/(333 mg) = 3 ml

Example: Ferrous sulfate (FESO4) is an iron supplement which comes in a liquid suspension with a concentration of 220 mg/5 ml. You are asked to give a dose of 100 mg. How many ml are needed to give this exact dose?

Set up the proportion: 220 mg/5 ml = 100 mg/x ml

Cross multiply to get this equation: (220 mg) (x ml) = (100 mg) (5 ml)

Solve for x by dividing both sides by 220 mg: x ml = (100 mg)(5 ml)/(220 mg) = 2.27 ml

Finding Total Volume in Concentrations

In most cases, prescription or medication orders will give you a total volume in the dispensing of a liquid formulation. In some cases, this information may not be given, so you will need to solve it yourself.

An example would be amoxicillin 250 mg/5 ml.

Directions: 100 mg po qid × 10 d

What is the total volume you want to give that will last the full ten days?

In this type of problem, you are given directions, which play a vital role in solving for the total volume needed. In all cases, the directions will be abbreviated, so knowledge of the most common abbreviations is necessary.

First of all, we do not know what the individual dose is as far as 100 mg, so our first step would be to solve for that.

Set up the proportion:	250 mg/5 ml = 100 mg/x ml
Cross multiply to get this equation:	(250 mg) (x ml) = (100 mg) (5 ml)
Solve for x by dividing both sides by 250 mg:	x ml = (100 mg)(5 ml)/(250 mg) = 2 ml

The next step would simply be to use your answer (dose), plug it into the directions, and multiply for total exact volume.

Directions: 100 mg by mouth four times a day for ten days

Understand that 100 mg is the same as 2 ml.

Directions: (2 ml) (4) (10) = 80 ml

Let's do another one:

FeSo4 220 mg/5 ml

Directions: 100 mg po qd × 60 d

What is the total volume you will give for this medication to last the full 60 days?

First step will be to find the individual dose:

Set up the proportion:	220 mg/5 ml = 100 mg/x ml
Cross multiply to get this equation:	(220 mg) (x ml) = (100 mg) (5 ml)
Solve for x by dividing both sides by 220 mg:	x ml = (100 mg)(5 ml)/(220 mg) = 2.27 ml

The next step would simply be to use your answer (dose), plug it into the given directions, and multiply to get the exact volume.

Directions: 100 mg by mouth once a day for 60 days

Understand that 100 mg is the same as 2.27 ml.

Directions: (2.27 ml) (1) (60) = 136.2 ml

Finding the Amount of Active Drug in a Container

In most cases, you will also see a number that follows the concentration, as in the following **example:**

EES 333 mg/5 ml 200 ml

The number 200 ml tells us the size of the container, or the total volume of medication we have on hand. This number is important in some problem solving, but is sometimes not used in other types of problem solving. In the case of the individual dose or total volume needed, this number is not used, unless the total volume needed is greater than the volume we have on hand.

This leads you to the understanding that it is important to know what information is necessary to solve your given problem and what information is not necessary. The national exams will give you numbers which are useful, but may not be necessary in the solving of specific types of problems.

When would you use the total volume on hand? You would use this information when the question asks for the total amount of active drug in your container.

Example: If you have amoxicillin 250 mg/5 ml 200 ml, how much total active drug is in this bottle?

To solve this, you need to know the concentration, and you also need to know total volume on hand.

Setup:	$250 \text{ mg}/5 \text{ ml} = x \text{ mg}/200 \text{ ml}$
Cross multiply to give this equation:	$(250 \text{ mg})(200 \text{ ml}) = (x \text{ mg})(5 \text{ ml})$
Solve for x by dividing both sides by 5:	$x \text{ mg} = (250 \text{ mg})(200 \text{ ml})/(x \text{ mg})(5 \text{ ml}) = 10{,}000 \text{ mg}$

Let's do another one:

You have ferrous sulfate 220 mg/5 ml 473 ml. How much total active drug is in this bottle?

To solve this, you need to know the concentration, and you also need to know total volume on hand.

Setup:	$220 \text{ mg}/5 \text{ ml} = x \text{ mg}/473 \text{ ml}$
Cross multiply to give this equation:	$(220 \text{ mg})(473 \text{ ml}) = (x \text{ mg})(5 \text{ ml})$
Solve for x by dividing both sides by 5:	$x \text{ mg} = (220 \text{ mg})(473 \text{ ml}) = (x \text{ mg})(5 \text{ ml}) = 20{,}812 \text{ mg}$

Let's do another one:

You have a cefaclor suspension 500 mg/5 ml 200 ml. How much total active drug is in this bottle?

Setup:	$500 \text{ mg}/5 \text{ ml} = x \text{ mg}/200 \text{ ml}$
Cross multiply to give this equation:	$(500 \text{ mg})(200 \text{ ml}) = (x \text{ mg})(5 \text{ ml})$
Solve for x by dividing both sides by 5:	$x \text{ mg} = (500 \text{ mg})(200 \text{ ml}) = (x \text{ mg})(5 \text{ ml}) = 20{,}000 \text{ mg}$

Use ratio and proportion for these concentrations, and see if you get the correct answers below:

a. You have a 250 mg/5 ml concentration of drug. How many ml are needed to give a dose of 400 mg?

b. Haloperidol comes in a strength of 2 mg/1 ml. How many ml are needed to give a dose of 6 mg?

c. Doxycylcine hyclate comes in a strength of 100 mg/5 ml. How many ml are needed to give a dose of 350 mg?

d. FeSO4 dose to be given is 500 mg. How many ml are needed if the concentration of liquid is 220 mg/5 ml?

e. If the concentration of drug is 400 mg/5 ml, how much drug will 12.5 ml give you?

Answers: a. 8 ml, b. 3 ml, c. 17.5 ml, d. 11.36 ml, e. 1,000 mg

Concentration and Compounding Problem Solving

Another type of problem solving where you would need the number/amount on hand is when the question asks how many tablets or capsules are needed to make a liquid concentration of a drug?

An example of this would be if a patient (let's call him Little Joey) cannot swallow a solid tablet, and there is no manufactured liquid formulation—how many tablets would you need to make a liquid formulation for Little Joey that will allow him to take his medication? In solving this type of problem, you will always be given a concentration and final volume needed.

Example: Little Joey has difficulty swallowing his 500 mg tablet of medication. The manufacturer does not make this medication in a liquid formulation, so the pharmacist will have to compound (prepare) this drug in a liquid formulation. How many 500 mg tablets are needed to make a 250 mg/5 ml 200 ml suspension or liquid formulation for Little Joey?

This will involve two parts:

Step 1: First, find the amount of active drug needed to make this liquid formulation.

Setup:	250 mg/5 ml = x mg/200 ml
Cross multiply to get this equation:	(250 mg) (200 ml) = (x mg) (5 ml)
Solve for x by dividing both sides by 5:	x mg = (250 mg) (200 ml) = (x mg) (5 ml) = 10,000 mg

Step 2: Set up a ratio and proportion to find how many tablets are needed.

Setup:	500 mg/1 tablet = 10,000 mg/x tablets
Solve for x by dividing both sides by 500 mg:	x tablets = (500 mg) (x tablets) = (1 tab) (10,000 mg) = 20 tablets

Therefore, 20 500 mg tablets will be ground using a mortar and pestle and will be incorporated with other ingredients to make a suspension of the drug that is 250 mg/5 ml 200 ml.

Let's do another one:

How many 200 mg capsules are needed to make a liquid concentration of 250 mg/5 ml 360 ml?

Step 1:

Setup:	250 mg/5 ml = x mg/360 ml
Cross multiply to get this equation:	(250 mg) (360 ml) = (x mg) (5 ml)
Solve for x by dividing both sides by 5:	x mg = (250 mg) (360 ml) = (x mg) (5 ml) = 18,000 mg

Step 2: Set up a ratio and proportion to find how many tablets are needed.

Setup:	200 mg/1 tablet = 18,000 mg/x tablets
Solve for x by dividing both sides by 200:	x tabs = (200 mg) (x tabs) = (1 tab) (18,000 mg) = 90 tablets

As mentioned before, ratio and proportion are used in many types of problem solving in the pharmacy setting and can easily be learned and mastered with practice. This chapter reviewed the use of ratio and proportion in problem solving that involves concentrations. The following chapter will use ratio and proportion for other types of problem solving as well.

Practice Questions

Answer the following multiple-choice questions with the best answer.

1. 1. What is the Arabic number for the following Roman numeral: CXXXIV
   a. 1,340
   b. 134
   c. 1,360
   d. 136

2. What is the Arabic number for the following Roman numeral: LXI
   a. 49
   b. 51
   c. 61
   d. 111

3. How many capsules need to be dispensed for the following prescription order:

   amoxicillin 250 mg, qty: XXVI

   a. 24
   b. 26
   c. 37
   d. 46

4. How many tabs will be used for one dose of a medication with the following directions?

   Directions: iv tabs po bid × 10d

   a. 1
   b. 2
   c. 3
   d. 4

5. Which fraction is smallest?
   a. $\frac{1}{16}$
   b. $\frac{1}{8}$
   c. $\frac{2}{16}$
   d. $\frac{3}{32}$

6. Which fraction is largest?
   a. $\frac{1}{12}$
   b. $\frac{3}{36}$
   c. $\frac{12}{72}$
   d. $\frac{5}{20}$

7. Reduce $\frac{21}{51}$ to lowest terms.
   a. $\frac{2}{5}$
   b. $\frac{3}{17}$
   c. $\frac{7}{17}$
   d. $\frac{21}{51}$

8. Reduce $\frac{36}{27}$ to lowest terms.
   a. $\frac{3}{4}$
   b. $\frac{4}{3}$
   c. $1\frac{1}{4}$
   d. $1\frac{1}{3}$

9. An oral antibiotic suspension makes 150 ml after reconstitution. Each dose is 5 ml. Each dose makes up what fractional part of the total?
   a. $\frac{1}{20}$
   b. $\frac{1}{30}$
   c. $\frac{1}{40}$
   d. $\frac{1}{50}$

10. A pharmacist had 4 oz of dextromethorphan HCl syrup in stock. She used $\frac{12}{4}$ oz to fill a prescription order. How much dextrome-othrphan HCl did she have left?
    a. $1\frac{3}{8}$ oz
    b. 1 oz
    c. $2\frac{5}{8}$ oz
    d. 2 oz

11. Express 25 thousandths in decimal form.
   a. 25,000
   b. 0.025
   c. 0.0025
   d. 0.,00025

12. Write $\frac{3}{20}$ as a decimal.
   a. 0.320
   b. 0.30
   c. 0.16
   d. 0.15

13. A clinical study of a new drug showed that the drug was effective in 586 of the 803 patients enrolled in the study. What is the decimal expression of the patients who benefited from the drug?
   a. $\frac{586}{803}$
   b. 73%
   c. 0.73
   d. $\frac{5}{8}$

14. Round 4.23891 to the nearest hundredth.
   a. 4.2389
   b. 4.239
   c. 4.24
   d. 4.23

15. Round 0.4912 to the nearest tenth.
   a. 0.491
   b. 0.49
   c. 0.4
   d. 0.5

16. Convert $\frac{5}{8}$ to a decimal.
   a. 0.58
   b. 0.158
   c. 0.125
   d. 0.625

17. Convert 0.16 to a fraction.
   a. $\frac{1}{16}$
   b. $\frac{1}{8}$
   c. $\frac{16}{50}$
   d. $\frac{4}{25}$

18. Which of the following is an incorrect way to state a proportion?
   a. a is to b as c is to d
   b. a:b = c:d
   c. $\frac{a}{b} = \frac{c}{d}$
   d. ab = cd

19. If a cough syrup contains 4 mg of chlorpheniramine in each 5 ml, how much chlorpheniramine (in milligrams) is contained in 240 ml of syrup?
   a. 24
   b. 48
   c. 96
   d. 192

20. Ferrous sulfate elixir contains 220 mg of ferrous sulfate per 5 ml. How much ferrous sulfate is in 473 ml of elixir?
   a. 1,100 mg
   b. 20,812 mg
   c. 94,600 mg
   d. 520,300 mg

21. If a potassium chloride solution contains 20 mg in each 15 ml, which volume of solution provides 35 mEq for the patient?
   a. 1.75 ml
   b. 8.57 ml
   c. 17.5 ml
   d. 26.25 ml

22. If a syringe contains 20 mg of medication in each 10 ml of solution, how many milligrams are administered to the patient when 3 ml is injected?
    a. 3 mg
    b. 4 mg
    c. 6 mg
    d. 12 mg

23. Which of the following ratio strength solutions is the most concentrated?
    a. 1:200
    b. 1:1,000
    c. 1:5,000
    d. 1:10,000

24. You have a bottle of Ceclor® with the concentration of 125 mg/5 ml. How many milliliters are needed to give this patient an exact 200 mg dose?
    a. 8 ml
    b. 10 ml
    c. 12.5 ml
    d. 15 ml

25. You have a bottle of prednisone 5 mg/5 ml. How many milliliters are needed to give this patient an exact 12 mg dose?
    a. 5 ml
    b. 6 ml
    c. 10 ml
    d. 12 ml

26. How much drug is needed to make a 1:100 120 ml solution?
    a. 5 g
    b. 6 g
    c. 10 g
    d. 12 g

27. Drug X has a concentration of 200 mg/5 ml 360 ml. What is the total amount of active drug in this bottle?
    a. 4,400 mg
    b. 14,400 mg
    c. 360 mg
    d. 24,000 mg

28. Drug X has a concentration of 125 mg/5 ml. How many milliliters are needed to give a 400 mg dose?
    a. 12 ml
    b. 14 ml
    c. 16 ml
    d. 18 ml

29. How many milliliters should you give for the following directions: 5 ml pot tid × 10d?
    a. 90 ml
    b. 150 ml
    c. 200 ml
    d. 360 ml

Use the following information to solve problems 30 and 31. Rx: Azithromycin 500 mg/5 ml 200 ml

Directions: 10 ml stat then 5 ml po bid × 20d

30. What does *200 ml* mean in this problem?
    a. number of doses in the prescription
    b. volume of medication on hand
    c. volume of active drug
    d. volume of inactive drug

31. How much active drug is in this container?
    a. 5,000 mg
    b. 10,000 mg
    c. 15,000 mg
    d. 20,000 mg

32. Mickey cannot swallow a 125 mg tablet, so the pharmacist is going to make a suspension of the medication that will have a concentration of 125 mg/5 ml 360 ml. How many tablets will be needed to prepare this suspension?
a. 60 tablets
b. 72 tablets
c. 80 tablets
d. 120 tablets

33. Mickey cannot swallow the 250 mg capsules either. How many 250 mg capsules will be needed to make the following suspension: Drug C 300 mg/5 ml 200 ml?
a. 24 capsules
b. 36 capsules
c. 48 capsules
d. 72 capsules

Use the following information to solve problem 34.

Rx: Doxycylcine Hyclate 100 mg/5 ml _____ ml

Directions: 10 ml stat then 5 ml po bid × 20d

34. How many milliliters are needed to fill this prescription?
a. 150 ml
b. 200 ml
c. 210 ml
d. 220 ml

Use the following information to solve problems 35 and 36.

Rx: Drug X is 0.4 g/5 ml 473 ml

Directions: 0.25 g po qid × 7d

35. What would the individual dose be?
a. approximately 2 ml
b. approximately 3 ml
c. approximately 4 ml
d. approximately 6 ml

36. What is the total volume of medication needed to last the full seven days?
a. approximately 56 ml
b. approximately 84 ml
c. approximately 112 ml
d. approximately 168 ml

37. You are asked to add meperidine HCl 10 mg to an IV of D5W 100 ml. Meperidine comes in a 4 ml vial with a concentration of 2 mg/1 ml. How much meperidine are you going to place in this IV bag?
a. 1 ml
b. 3 ml
c. 5 ml
d. 10 ml

38. You have an injectable drug with the concentration of 25 mg/2.5 ml 10 ml and are asked to prepare a syringe with a dose of 12 mg in it. What will the volume of your syringe be?
a. 0.8 ml
b. 1.2 ml
c. 1.8 ml
d. 2 ml

Use the following information to solve problems 39 and 40.

Rx: Drug D 325 mg/5 ml _____ ml
Directions: 580 mg po bid × 30d

39. What would the individual dose be?
a. approximately 4 ml
b. approximately 7 ml
c. approximately 9 ml
d. approximately 12 ml

40. What is the total volume needed for this prescription to last the full 30 days?
a. approximately 240 ml
b. approximately 420 ml
c. approximately 540 ml
d. approximately 720 ml

Answers and Explanations

1. b. CXXXIV: $100 + 10 + 10 + 10 + 4 = 134$

2. c. LXI: $50 + 10 + 1 = 61$

3. b. XXVI: $10 + 10 + 5 + 1 = 26$

4. d. Four tablets, as IV = 4

5. a. $\frac{1}{16}$ is the smallest of the fractions presented.

6. d. $\frac{5}{20} = \frac{1}{4}$ is the largest of the fractions presented.

7. c. Divide both 21 and 51 by 3 to get 7 and 17.

8. d. $\frac{36}{27} = 1\frac{9}{27} = 1\frac{1}{3}$

9. b. Set up the ratio and reduce the fraction:
$$\frac{5\ ml}{150\ ml} = \frac{5\ ml}{150 ml} = \frac{5}{150} = \frac{1}{30}$$

10. b. $\frac{12}{4}$ oz = 3 oz dispensed, which leaves 1 oz left from the original 4 oz container.

11. c. The first decimal place to the right of the decimal point is tenths, the second place is hundredths, and the third place is thousandths.

12. d. 3 divided by 20 equals 0.15.

13. c. 586 divided by 803 = 0.73; $\frac{586}{803}$ is incorrect because it is not a decimal.

14. c. Hundredths is the second decimal place; the numeral in the thousandths place is 5 or greater, so you round 3 in the hundredths place up to 4, and the subsequent decimal places are dropped.

15. d. Tenths is the first decimal place; the numeral in the hundredths place is 5 or greater, so you round the 4 in the tenths place up to 5, and the subsequent decimal places are dropped.

16. d. 5 divided by 8 is 0.625.

17. d. $0.16 = \frac{16}{100}$; reduce the fraction by dividing each number by 4 to get $\frac{4}{25}$.

18. d. A proportion is two equal ratios. Both ab and cd are products, not ratios. Each of the other expressions is an equation of two ratios.

19. d. You solve this problem by setting up the proportion 4 mg/5 ml = x mg/240 ml. Then solve the proportion: (4 mg)(240 ml) = (x mg)(5 ml), x = (4 mg)(240 ml)/(5 ml) = 192 ml.

20. b. Solve this problem the same way as the previous one: set up the proportion 220 mg/5 ml = x mg/473 ml, and solve for x. In this case, x = (220 mg)(473 ml)/(5 ml) = 20,812 mg.

21. d. Again use proportion to find the answer: 20 m Eq/15 ml = 35 mEq/x ml, and solve for x. x = (35 mEq × 15 ml)/(20 ml) = 26.25 ml.

22. c. Again use proportion to find the answer: 20 mg/10 ml = x mg/3 ml, and solve for x. x = (20 mg)(3 ml)/(10 ml) = 6 ml.

23. a. This would be most concentrated, as there is 1 g of active drug per 200 ml solution.

24. a. Again, use proportion to find the answer: 125 mg/5 ml = 200 mg/x ml, and solve for x. x = (200 mg)(5 ml)/(125 mg) = 8 ml.

25. d. 5 mg/5 ml = 12 mg/x ml, and solve for x. x = (12 mg)(5 ml)/(5 mg) = 12 ml.

26. d. A ratio strength of 1:100 is the same as 1 g per 100 ml or 1 g/100 ml. So how many g are in 120 ml? 1 g/100 ml = x g/120 ml, and solve for x. x = (1 g)(120 ml)/(100 g) = 12 g.

27. b. 200 mg/5 ml 360 ml setup would be: x = (200 mg)(360 ml) = (x mg)(5 ml) = 14,400 mg.

28. c. x = 125 mg/5 ml = 400 mg/x ml = 16 ml.

29. b. Simply plug 5 ml into your directions and multiply: (5 ml)(3 times a day)(10 days) = 150 ml.

30. b. When a number follows a concentration, it indicates the volume of medication or drug you have on hand.

31. d. x = (500 mg)(200 ml)/(5 ml) = 20,000 mg.

32. b. First, figure out how much total drug is needed: x = (125 mg)(360 ml)/(5 ml) = 9,000 mg, then divide the total dose needed by the strength of the individual tablet: (9,000 mg)/(125 mg) = 72 tablets.

33. c. Solve the same way as question 32: x = (300 mg)(200 ml)/(5 ml) = 12,000 mg, (12,000 mg/250 mg) = 48 capsules.

34. c. From the directions, you can tell what total volume is needed. 10 ml now, then (5 ml)(2)(20) = 210 ml.

35. b. $(0.4 \text{ g})(x \text{ ml}) = (0.25 \text{ g})(5 \text{ ml})$; $x = (0.25 \text{ g})(5 \text{ ml})/(0.4 \text{ g}) = 3.13 \text{ ml}$, or approximately 3 ml.

36. b. $x = (3 \text{ ml})(4)(7) = 84 \text{ ml}$.

37. c. $(2 \text{ mg})(x \text{ ml}) = (10 \text{ mg})(1 \text{ ml})$; $x = (10 \text{ mg})(1 \text{ ml})/(2 \text{ mg}) = 5 \text{ ml}$.

38. b. $(25 \text{ mg})(x \text{ ml}) = (12 \text{ mg})(2.5 \text{ ml})$; $x = (12 \text{ mg})(2.5 \text{ ml})/(25 \text{ mg}) = 1.2 \text{ ml}$.

39. c. $(325 \text{ mg})(x \text{ ml}) = (580 \text{ mg})(5 \text{ ml})$; $x = (580 \text{ mg})(5 \text{ ml})/(325 \text{ mg}) = 8.9 \text{ ml}$, or approximately 9 ml.

40. c. $x = (9 \text{ ml})(2)(30) = 540 \text{ ml}$.

CHAPTER

10 ▶ Pharmacy Math II

CHAPTER OVERVIEW

The last chapter was a basic overview of Roman numerals and fractions, as well as an introduction to ratio, proportion, and concentrations using those concepts. In this chapter, we will review different systems used in calculations and continue with different types of pharmacy calculations using, again, ratio and proportion. Included will be conversion problems, where we will be asked to go equate one unit of measurement to another. This type of problem solving is essential in dosage calculations.

TERMS

apothecary	kilo-
cubic centimeter	liter
equivalent	meter
grain	metric
gram	micro-
gallon	milli-
household	unit
international unit	

In order to safely prepare and accurately dispense the prescribed amount of medications to patients, you must be familiar with dosage calculations. A knowledge of the weights and measures used in the prescription and administration of medications is necessary. The systems of weights and measures used by health professionals, as discussed in the previous chapter, is mainly the **metric** system of measurement. There are other systems used in the pharmacy setting as well, such as the **apothecary**, avoirdupois, and **household** systems. Conversions between these systems will be discussed in this chapter.

This chapter reviews the fundamentals of measurement by weight, volume, length, temperature, and also reviews application of measurement systems commonly used in pharmacy practice. Examples will demonstrate critical concepts, while problem sets will evaluate your competency in these areas. To become a skilled pharmacy technician, you will need a basic understanding of these measurement systems and the ability to use them in daily practice.

The Metric System

The metric system (also known as the International System of Units, or SI) was introduced in France in 1791, legalized in the United States in 1866, and is the most widely used system of measurement in the world. Despite the fact that it became a legal standard in the United States in the nineteenth century, it is still not in universal usage in this country. In fact, the United States remains one of a tiny number of countries that have not adopted the metric system. However, it is the predominant system in use for scientific studies and the practice of healthcare.

The accuracy and simplicity of the metric system lie in the fact that it is based on the decimal system, in which everything is measured in multiples or fractions of ten.

For this reason, metric numbers are expressed as whole numbers or decimal numbers. See the chart below for a comparison of how each unit of measure compares to another.

PREFIX	SYMBOL	VALUE	WEIGHT	VOLUME	LENGTH
kilo-	k	1,000	kilogram (kg)		kilometer (km)
hecto-	h	100			
deka-	da	10			
BASE	–	1	gram (g)	liter (L)	meter (m)
deci-	d	0.1		deciliter (dL)	
centi-	c	0.01			centimeter (cm)
milli-	m	0.001	milligram (mg)	milliliter (mL or ml)	millimeter (mm)
micro-	mc	0.,000001	microgram (mcg)	microliter (mcL)	micrometer (mcm)

Standard Measures

In the metric system, the standard measure for length is the **meter** (m). A meter is 1/10,000,000 of the distance from the North Pole to the equator (and is slightly longer than one yard). This measure of length is commonly used to express a patient's height and determine growth patterns. It is not used directly to calculate doses.

The standard measure for weight is the **gram** (g), defined as the weight of one **cubic centimeter** (cc) of distilled water at 4°C. Dry medications are measured in units of weight. A patient's weight is measured in kilograms, which is equal to 1,000 grams. Often, doses of drugs are based on a patient's weight.

The standard measure for volume is the **liter** (L), defined as the volume of 1,000 cubic centimeters (about one quart). Liquid medications are measured in units of volume. The liter and milliliter (mL or ml = 1/1,000th of a liter) are used to calculate concentrations of solutions when determining doses.

Liquid volume is measured in liters or milliliters:

Largest Number ⟶ Smallest Number

liter is L   milliliter is ml

1 L = 1,000 ml

The measure of weight is a little bit more involved:

Largest Number ⟶ Smallest Number

kilogram is kg   gram is g   milligram is mg   microgram is mcg

In the metric system, the unit or abbreviation always follows the numeric amount (e.g., 2 mg, 25 ml, or 5.6 g). Decimal fractions are used to designate fractional amounts.

The following are units of measure you will see in pharmacy.

Length

Standard length is the meter (m).

$$1 \text{ centimeter (cm)} = \tfrac{1}{100} \text{ th of a meter (0.01 m)}$$

Volume

Standard volume is the liter (L).

1 liter = 1,000 milliliters

1 milliliter = 1/1,000th of a liter (0.001 L)

Note that the cubic centimeter (cc) is another way of expressing volume. A cubic centimeter is the amount of space occupied by one milliliter of water at 4°C, but you may see the abbreviations cc and ml used interchangeably.

Weight

Standard weight is the gram (g).

  1 kilogram = 1,000 grams

  1 gram = 1,000 milligrams

  1 milligram = 1/1,000th of a gram (0.001 g)

  1 microgram = 1/1,000,000th of a gram (0.,000001 g)

Note that microgram is sometimes mistakenly abbreviated as "μg," and gram is abbreviated as "Gm" or "gm." You should learn and use only the standardized abbreviations as listed above.

The Apothecary System

Apothecary is another name for a pharmacy, commonly used in Europe. The apothecary system of measure is also called the wine measure, or the U.S. liquid measure system. This is an archaic system left over from the Middle Ages, but some practitioners may still use it in writing prescription/medication orders because that is the way they learned it. It may also be used to designate doses for medications that have existed for years. It is slowly being replaced by the metric system, but until prescribers adopt the metric system of measures exclusively, you will have to know at least one unit of measure in the apothecary system.

The unit of measurement that you should know is the **grain** (gr), which is approximately **equivalent** to 60 mg.

APOTHECARY MEASURE		
Unit	Abbreviation	Approximate Equivalent
grain	gr	60 mg

Unlike the metric system, in which the unit follows the numeric quantity, in the apothecary system, the measure or its abbreviation precedes the value. For example, three grains is written gr iii instead of iii gr.

Standard Measures
Weight

In the apothecary system, the standard measure for weight is the grain. The origin of this term is unknown, but it is thought that at one time, solids were measured by using grains of wheat as the standard. There are a few familiar drugs still dispensed in grains: aspirin or acetaminophen (gr v or gr x), phenobarbital sodium (gr $\frac{1}{4}$, $\frac{1}{2}$, i), and nitroglycerin (gr $\frac{1}{150}$, gr $\frac{1}{200}$).

The Household System

The household system is the most commonly used system in outpatient settings, where a patient measures liquids at home without accurate measuring equipment. The home measuring equipment usually consists of commonly used home utensils (teaspoons, tablespoons, cups, etc.). It is the least accurate of the systems of measure and should not be used to determine doses of drugs. However, you should be familiar with the household system of measurement so you can explain take-home prescription directions at the time of dispensing and ensure that the prescription label includes directions that will be understood by the patient—including what volume of medication to take. The following table shows the basic units of this system. Since teaspoons, tablespoons, and cups vary from household to household, it is obvious why this system is not completely accurate for measuring medications.

HOUSEHOLD MEASURES			
UNIT	ABBREVIATION	APPROXIMATE EQUIVALENTS IN OTHER SYSTEMS	APPROXIMATE MEASUREMENT* (EXACT IN PARENTHESES)
drop	gtt	n/a	n/a
teaspoonful	tsp	3 tsp = 1 tbsp	5 ml
tablespoonful	tbsp	1 tbsp = 3 tsp	15 ml
ounce (liquid)	fl oz	1 fl oz = 2 tbsp	30 ml (29.57 ml)
ounce (weight)	oz	16 oz = 1 lb	30 g (28.35 g)
cup	c	1 c = 8 fl oz	240 ml
pint	pt	1 pt = 2 c	480 ml (473 ml)
quart	qt	1 qt = 2 pt = 4 c	1 L (946 ml)
gallon	gal	1 gal = 4 qt = 8 pt	3,785 ml
pound	lb	1 lb = 16 oz	480 g (454 g)

*For the national exam, it is okay to use approximate measurements.

Note that people commonly use the term *drop* when referring to measuring medications. Use caution when working with this measure, especially with potent medications, because the volume of a drop depends not only on the viscosity (thickness) of the liquid, but also on the size, shape, and way the dropper is held and used. To measure small amounts of liquid accurately, use a 1 ml syringe (with fractional milliliter marks) instead of a dropper. Eye drops are an exception to this rule; the calibrated dropper included with the drug delivers a correctly sized droplet.

Special Units of Measure for Medications

Some medications are measured in special units. The medications that use these measurements are prescribed, prepared, and administered using the same system. This eliminates the need to learn how to convert these units into another system.

A **unit** is the amount of medication required to produce a certain effect. The size of the unit varies for each drug. Some medications, such as vitamins, are measured in standardized units called **international units**. Medications that are ordered in units will also be labeled in units. A milliunit is 1,000th of a unit.

Some drugs are measured in milliequivalents (mEq), which is a unit of measure based on the chemical combining power of a substance. Electrolytes are commonly measured in milliequivalents.

The three most common special units are described in the following table.

UNIT NAME	DESCRIPTION	USE
international unit	represents a unit of potency	measuring vitamins and chemicals
unit	represents a standardized amount needed to produce a desired effect	measuring medications which include heparin, insulin, and penicillin
milliequivalent (mEq)	represents a unit of measure specifically for electrolytes, which are elements on the periodic table that carry a positive or negative charge	describing concentration of electrolytes such as calcium, magnesium, potassium, and sodium

Aside from understanding that there are three common special units, as a pharmacy technician you need not understand their significance except that these are the units of measure for specific medications. Although there are conversions involved with these units in the pharmacy setting, they are done by the pharmacist—and this will not be asked of you on the national exam.

Conversions and Equivalencies between Systems

In conversion, or the changing of one unit of measure to another unit of measure such that they are equal, can easily be solved using ratios and proportions. In Chapter 6 you were taught what a ratio is and that a proportion is two equal ratios. If you recall, your setup was always about what information you "have" equal to information you "want."

have = want

You were also instructed on how to solve concentration type of problem solving using the ratio and proportion method, and always using the concentration as information you "have."

For conversions, it is important that you memorize at least these ten equivalencies, as the national exam will not give them to you.

- 1 Kg = 1,000 g
- 1 Kg = 2.2 lb (pounds)
- 1 L = 1,000 ml
- 1 g = 1,000 mg
- 1 mg = 1,000 mcg

- 1 gr = 60 mg
- 1 oz = 30 g or 30 ml
- 1 tsp = 5 ml
- 1 lb = 454 g
- 1 tbsp = 15 ml

Approximate equivalents are used for conversions from one system to another. They describe approximately how much of a unit in one system it takes to equal a unit in another system. Identifying the equivalent is the necessary first step in a conversion.

Solving Conversions Using Ratio and Proportion

Converting from one unit of measure to another unit of measure can be done easily, using ratio and proportion.

Example: How many milliliters are in 3 liter solution?

As you recall, the first step involved in the solving of concentration type problem solving was to indicate the concentration as information you "have," and then from there create your proportion and solve it using the steps you've already learned.

In solving conversions, your first step is to indicate what your two units have in common from the list of ten conversions you memorized, and then use this as information you have in setting up your proportion.

From the list of ten conversions, you find the units ml and L have the following in common: 1 L is equal to 1,000 ml, or 1 L = 1,000 ml. This will be the information you have in your setup.

Set up the proportion:

1 L/1,000 ml = 3 L/x ml

Remember: What you have in common from your list of ten conversions is what you "have."

Cross multiply to get this equation:	(1 L) (x ml) = (3 L) (1,000 ml)
Solve for x by dividing both sides by 1:	x ml = (3 L)(1,000 ml)/(1 L) = 3,000 ml

Let's try another one:

How many milligrams are there in 32 grains?

Set up the proportion:	1 gr/60 mg = 32 gr/x mg
Cross multiply to get this equation:	(1 gr) (x mg) = (32 gr) (60 mg)
Solve for x by dividing both sides by 1:	x mg = (32 gr) (60 mg)/(1) = 1,920 mg

Let's try another one:

456 milliliters is equal to how many liters?

Set up the proportion:	1 L/1,000 ml = x L/456 ml
Cross multiply to get this equation:	(1 L) (456 ml) = (x L) (1,000 ml)
Solve for x by dividing both sides by 1,000:	x L = (1 L) (456 ml)/(1,000) = 0.456 L, or 0.46 L if we reduce to the hundredths place.

What if we have a conversion in which one of our ten memorized conversions is not available? In most cases, we can still solve the conversion, but will have to do it in several steps, also known as multistep conversion problem solving.

Example: 45 ounces are equal to how many liters?

As you can see, one of our ten memorized conversions does not involve converting liters to ounces or vice versa. This is not a problem, as we can still use our ten conversions, but will need to create a link for our beginning unit of measure to our ending unit of measure. In other words, how do you get from ounces to liters?

In the list of ten conversions, we have ounces to milliliters, We can use this, creating a link from ounces to milliliters and then liters. oz → ml → L

Step 1: Convert 45 ounces to x milliliters (oz → ml).

Set up the proportion:	1 oz/30 ml = 45 oz/x ml
Cross multiply to get this equation:	(1 oz) (x ml) = (45 oz) (30 ml)
Solve for x by dividing both sides by 1:	x ml = (45 oz)(30 ml)/(1) = 1,350 ml

However, you are not looking for milliliters. You are are looking for liters.

Step 2: Convert 1,350 milliliters to liters (ml → L).

Set up the proportion:	1 L/1,000 ml = x L/1,350 ml
Cross multiply to get this equation:	(1 L) (1,350 ml) = (x L) (1,000 ml)
Solve for x by dividing both sides by 1,000:	x L = (1 L) (1,350 ml)/(1,000) = 1.3 L

As you can see, the ten conversions will solve 95% of conversion type problems, not only on the national exam, but in the pharmacy setting as well!

Let's try another one:

Example: 34.5 kilograms is equal to how many ounces?

Your created link: kg → g → oz

Step 1:

Set up the proportion:	1 kg/1,000 g = 34.5 kg/x g
Cross multiply to get this equation:	(1 kg) (x g) = (34.5 kg) (1,000 g)
Solve for x by dividing both sides by 1:	x g = (34. 5 kg) (1,000 g)/(1) = 34,500 g

But we are not looking for grams, we are looking for milligrams.

Step 2: Convert 34,500 grams to ounces (g → oz).

Setup the proportion: 1 oz/30 g = x oz/34,500 g

Cross multiply to get this equation: (1 oz) (34,500 g) = (x oz) (30 g)

Solve for x by dividing both sides by 30: x oz = (1 oz) (34,500 g)/(30) = 1,150 oz

Convert the following units using ratio and proportion, and see if you get the correct answer below:

a. 450 g = x mg
b. 24 L = x ml
c. 63.4 gr = x mg
d. 1.5 L = x ml
e. 567 mg = x g

Answers: **a.** 450,000 mg, **b.** 24,000 ml, **c.** 3,804 mg, **d.** 1,500 ml, **e.** 0.57 g

Weight and Individual Dose Conversions

Today, the dosing of medication is done by kilogram body weight, which can be found in your reference books, literature, or drug inserts. Although a few review books will go over different rules, such as Young's, Clarke's, and Fred's rules in dosing, these are archaic and not used today in the pharmacy setting, and this will not be on the national exam.

An example of dosing by body weight in kilograms would be: 10 mg/kg body weight. If there is no number in front of the unit, the unit is always 1; so the correct dose would be: 10 mg/1 kg body weight.

Example: Little Joey weighs 64 lb and is to be given a dose of medication of 10 mg/kg body weight. How many milligrams of drug are we going to give Little Joey?

Set up the proportion: 10 mg/kg = x mg/64 lb

In this case, what you have and want is given in your problem.

When you create a proportion, the units on top (numerator) on both sides must be equal, as well as the units on bottom (denominator) on both sides. We see mg in both numerators, but in the denominators we see kg and lb, so they do not match. You must make them match by converting either lb to kg or kg to lb so they will match. I always suggest changing kg to lb, as this is one of your ten conversions: 1 kg = 2.2 lb

New setup: 10 mg/2.2 lb = x mg/64 lb

Now the units match and we can go ahead and solve!

Cross multiply to get this equation: (10 mg) (64 lb) = (x mg) (2.2 lb)

Solve for x by dividing both sides by 2.2: x mg = (10 mg) (64 lb)/(2.2) = 290.91 mg

If we were given the same problem and were given a concentration of drug, we could easily solve how much drug to dispense as well.

Example: Little Joey weighs 64 lb and is to be given a dose of medication of 10 mg/kg body weight. We also have the medication for Little Joey that is 100 mg/5 ml 473 ml. How many milliliters of medication would we give Little Joey?

The first step would be simply to find out what dose is needed for Little Joey, which we did previously and came up with the answer: 290.01 mg.

The second step would be similar to the problems discussed in Chapter 9.

Set up the proportion: have = want

If you see a concentration in your problem, this will be what you "have" in setting up your proportion!

100 mg/5 ml = 290.1 mg/x ml

What you want is the dose you came up with for Little Joey.

Cross multiply to get this equation: (100 mg) (x ml) = (290.1 mg) (5 ml)

Solve for x by dividing both sides by 100: x ml = (290.1 mg) (5 ml)/(100) = 14.51 ml

Practice Questions

1. 150 mg is how many grams?
   a. 0.0015
   b. 0.015
   c. 0.15
   d. 1.5

2. 2,250 ml is how many liters?
   a. 0.0225
   b. 0.225
   c. 2.25
   d. 22.5

3. Which of the following is NOT an official metric/SI abbreviation?
   a. L
   b. g
   c. gr
   d. kg

4. An inhalation aerosol contains 150 mg of metaproterenol sulfate, which is sufficient for 200 inhalations. How many micrograms are in each inhalation?
   a. 75
   b. 750
   c. 133
   d. 1,330

5. A liquid contains 0.25 mg of drug per milliliter. How many milligrams of the drug are in 1.5 L?
   a. 0.375
   b. 3.75
   c. 37.5
   d. 375

6. Add 0.025 kg, 1,780 mg, 2.65 g, and 755 mcg and express the answer in grams.
   a. 2,537.675
   b. 1,807.7255
   c. 29.430755
   d. 27.652535

7. Of the following metric system unit lists, which one would be in the correct order from largest weight to smallest weight?
   a. g to mg to mcg to kg
   b. kg to g to mg to mcg
   c. mcg to mg to g to kg
   d. kg to mcg to mg to g

8. Children's chewable aspirin tablets contain $1\frac{1}{4}$ gr of aspirin in each tablet. How many milligrams is this in each tablet?
   a. 60
   b. 75
   c. 180
   d. 325

9. 1/200 gr of the drug is equal to how many milligrams?
   a. 0.15
   b. 0.2
   c. 0.3
   d. 0.4

10. Approximately how many pints of cough syrup can be filled from 1 gal of cough syrup?
   a. 4
   b. 8
   c. 12
   d. 16

11. How many gr ss codeine capsules can be made from 120 mg of codeine powder?

   a. 2

   b. 4

   c. 6

   d. 8

12. How many teaspoons are in one tablespoon?

   a. $\frac{1}{3}$

   b. 1

   c. 3

   d. 5

13. How many cups are in one gallon?

   a. 8

   b. 16

   c. 24

   d. 32

14. How many teaspoons are in 2 oz of liquid?

   a. 6

   b. 12

   c. 24

   d. 30

15. The pharmacist dispenses 180 ml from an unopened 480 ml container of suspension. How many ounces are left over in the container?

   a. 6

   b. 8

   c. 10

   d. 12

16. gr ii is equal to how many milligrams?

   a. 30

   b. 45

   c. 60

   d. 120

17. 90 lb is equal to how many kilograms?

   a. 40.91

   b. 45

   c. 180

   d. 198

18. 1 gal is equal to how many milliliters?

   a. 360

   b. 480

   c. 1,000

   d. 3,785

19. One teaspoon is equal to how many milliliters?

   a. 3

   b. 4

   c. 5

   d. 6

20. 180 ml is equal to how many fluid ounces?

   a. 2

   b. 4

   c. 6

   d. 8

21. 456 ml is equal to how many liters?

   a. 0.456

   b. 4.56

   c. 45.6

   d. 456

22. 45 ml is equal to how many tablespoons?

   a. 2

   b. 3

   c. 4

   d. 5

23. A physician advises a patient to take a baby aspirin tablet (75 mg) to reduce the risk of heart attack. The patient decides to cut a five grain (gr v) tablet into doses. How many doses can be obtained from each tablet?
    a. 4
    b. 6
    c. 8
    d. 10

24. Using household measure, how would you instruct a patient to take 5 ml of decongestant syrup?
    a. Take one tablespoonful.
    b. Take two tablespoonsful.
    c. Take one teaspoonful.
    d. Take one ounce.

25. Using household measure, how would you tell a patient to take 60 ml of a liquid?
    a. Take one teaspoonful.
    b. Take two teaspoonsful.
    c. Take three teaspoonsful.
    d. Take four tablespoonsful.

26. A pharmacist received a prescription calling for 30 capsules, each to contain 1/200 gr of nitroglycerin. How many 0.4 mg nitroglycerin tablets would supply the amount required?
    a. 5
    b. 11
    c. 22.5
    d. 45

27. An antianemia tablet contains 300 mg of ferrous sulfate, which is equivalent to 60 mg of elemental iron. How many grains each of ferrous sulfate and elemental iron will the patient receive from one tablet?
    a. 2.5 and $\frac{1}{2}$
    b. 5 and 1
    c. 10 and 2
    d. 12 and $2\frac{1}{2}$

28. 34.5 kg is equal to how many ounces?
    a. 340
    b. 960
    c. 1,150
    d. 1,420

29. If one fluid ounce of cough syrup contains ten grains of sodium citrate, how much sodium citrate (in milligrams) is contained in 5 ml?
    a. 16.67
    b. 33
    c. 45
    d. 78

30. A formula for a cough syrup contains gr xviii of codeine phosphate per teaspoonful. How many grams of codeine phosphate should be used in preparing one pint of the cough syrup?
    a. 480
    b. 172.8
    c. 111.98
    d. 1,728

Use the following information to solve problems 31 and 32.

An oral suspension of vancomycin 500 mg/5 ml 473 ml is prescribed for a patient who weighs 214 lb. The literature indicates the dose to be 8 mg/kg body weight.

31. What dose is needed for this patient?
    a. approximately 540 mg
    b. approximately 778 mg
    c. approximately 995 mg
    d. approximately 1,260 mg

32. How many milliliters of vancomycin are you going to give this patient?
    a. approximately 5.4 ml
    b. approximately 7.8 ml
    c. approximately 10 ml
    d. approximately 12 ml

33. If 100 mg of heparin is equivalent to 4,500 units, how many grains are required to obtain one unit?
a. 0.075
b. 0.75
c. 7.5
d. 2,700

34. How many milligrams are in 10 grains of aspirin?
a. 300
b. 325
c. 600
d. 750

35. If the literature with a medication states a dose should be 0.04 g/kg body weight, how many milligrams of medication would be given to a patient who weighs 124 lb?
a. 960 mg
b. 1,480 mg
c. 1,856 mg
d. 2,255 mg

Use the following information to solve problems 36, 37, and 38.

FeSO4 220 mg/5 ml 473 ml

Directions: 120 mg po bid × 120d

36. How much total active drug is in this container?
a. 14.5 g
b. 16.2 g
c. 18.4 g
d. 20.8 g

37. How many milliliters should you give this patient for one dose?
a. 1.6
b. 2.7
c. 3.4
d. 5.2

38. Does this container have enough medication to last the full 120 days? If not, how many days will this medication last?
a. There is enough medication to last the full 120 days.
b. This medication will last approximately 60 days.
c. This medication will last approximately 90 days.
d. This medication will last approximately 110 days.

39. If there are 3 ml of the drug paregoric in each tablespoonful of medication, how many milliliters of paregoric would you find in one teaspoonful of medication?
a. 1 ml
b. 1.2 ml
c. 2 ml
d. 2.2 ml

40. If the cost of one-half ounce of zinc oxide is $3.45, what is the cost of 120 g?
a. $12.20
b. $16.40
c. $24.10
d. $27.60

Answers and Explanations

1. c. There are 1,000 mg per 1 g. Setup: 1 g/1,000 mg = x g/150 mg; (1 g) (150 mg)/(1,000 mg) = 0.15 g.

2. c. There are 1,000 ml per liter; therefore, 2,250 ml is equivalent to 2.25 L.

3. c. Grain (gr) is not part of the metric system, but rather the apothecary system.

4. b. 150 mg equals 150,000 mcg; 150,000 mcg divided by 200 inhalations is 750 mcg per inhalation.

5. d. 1.5 L equals 1,500 ml. Setup: (0.25 mg)/(1 ml) = (x mg)/(1,500 ml); x = 375 mg.

6. c. In order to add different values correctly, they must each be converted to the same units before adding. 0.025 kg = 25 g, 1,780 mg = 1.78 g, and 755 mcg = 0.000755 g; therefore, 25 g + 1.78 g + 2.65 g + 0.000755 g = 29.430755 g.

7. b. Kg to g to mg to mcg would be the correct answer, as each one is a multiple of 1,000. For example: 1 kg = 1,000 g, 1 g = 1,000 mg, 1 mg = 1,000 mcg.

8. b. $1\frac{1}{4}$ gr is the same as gr 1.25. Setup: (1 gr)/(60 mg) = (1.25 gr)/(x mg) = 75 mg. Note: Realize that this is the approximate conversion, as the exact conversion would be 64.8 mg, and the answer would be 81 mg. But for exam purposes, we can use approximate units of measure. Answers on the national exam will be far enough apart to know if you have the correct answer or not, whether using approximate or exact conversions.

9. c. 1/200 gr needs to be changed to a decimal number by dividing the top number (numerator) by the bottom number (denominator): 1/200 = 0.005. Now you can use this number in your setup: (1 gr)/(60 mg) = (0.005 gr)/(x mg) = 0.3 mg

10. b. There are eight pints in one gallon.

11. b. Ss means one-half (0.5) and 0.5 gr = 30 mg; (1 cap)/(0.5 gr) = (x cap)/(120 mg) = 4 capsules.

12. c. One teaspoonful equals 5 ml; one tablespoonful equals 15 ml; 15 ml divided by 5 ml equals 3.

13. b. There are eight pints per gallon and two cups per pint; therefore, there are 16 cups per gallon.

14. b. One fluid ounce equals 30 ml, so two fluid ounces equal 60 ml. One teaspoonful equals 5 ml; 60 ml divided by 5 ml per teaspoonful = 12 teaspoonsful.

15. c. 480 ml minus 180 ml = 300 ml. Setup: (1 oz)/(30 ml) = (x oz)/(300 ml); x = 10 oz.

16. d. There are 60 mg per grain; therefore, gr ii is equal to 120 mg.

17. a. There are 2.2 pounds per kilogram; therefore, 90 pounds divided by 2.2 pounds per kilogram is equal to 40.91 kg. Reminder setup: (1 kg/2.2 lb) = (x kg/90 lb).

18. d. There are 3,785 ml in 1 gallon.

19. c. There are 5 ml per teaspoonful.

20. c. There are 30 ml per fluid ounce; therefore, 180 ml divided by 30 ml per fluid ounce equals six fluid ounces.

21. a. Setup: (1 L)/(1,000 ml) = (x L)/(456 ml); x = 0.456 L, or 0.47 L if we round off to the hundredths place.

22. b. There are 15 ml per tablespoonful; therefore, 45 ml divided by 15 ml per tablespoonful equals three tablespoonsful.

23. a. A five grain tablet contains 300 mg; if you divide the tablet into quarters, each piece will contain 75 mg. So there are four doses in a five-grain tablet.

24. c. There are 5 ml per teaspoonful.

25. d. There are 15 ml per tablespoonful; therefore, 60 ml divided by 15 ml per tablespoonful equals four tablespoonsful.

26. c. 30 capsules, multiplied by 1/200 grain per capsule equals 0.15 grains. There are 60 mg per grain, so 0.15 grains equals 9 mg. 9 mg divided by 0.4 mg per tablet equals 22.5 tablets.

27. b. One grain = 60 mg. Therefore, 300 mg divided by 60 mg per grain equals five grains, and 60 mg divided by 60 mg per grain equals one grain.

28. c. This is a multistep conversion: kg → g → oz. Solve for grams first then from that answer, find out how many ounces.

29. a. There are 30 ml in one fluid ounce, so if there are 10 grains in 30 ml, there are 0.3333 grains per milliliter. 0.33 grains per milliliter multiplied by 5 ml equals 16.67 mg.

30. c. One pint equals 480 ml; one teaspoonful equals 5 ml. Therefore, there are 96 teaspoonsful per pint. 96 teaspoonsful times 18 grains per teaspoonful equals 1,728 grains. There are 15.432 grains per gram. So 1,728 grains divided by 15.432 grains per gram equals 111.98 g. We use the exact conversion in this case, because codeine is a potent drug.

31. b. Realize 1 kg is equal to 2.2 lb. Setup: $(8 \text{ mg})/(2.2 \text{ lb}) = (x \text{ mg})/(214 \text{ lb})$. $x = 778.18$ mg.

32. b. Setup: $(500 \text{ mg})/(5 \text{ ml}) = (778.18 \text{ mg})/(x \text{ ml})$; $x = 7.78$ ml.

33. b. 4,500 units divided by 100 mg equals 45 units per milligram. There are 60 mg per grain and 45 units per milligram divided by 60 mg per grain, which equals 0.75 units per grain.

34. c. There are 60 mg per grain. Therefore, there are 600 mg in 10 grains. This is an approximate conversion.

35. d. First, you need to find out how many milligrams 0.4 g is. Once you determine that it is 400 mg, then we can set up our problem with the understanding that 1 kg is equal to 2.2 lb. Setup: $(400 \text{ mg})/(2.2 \text{ lb}) = (x \text{ mg})/(124 \text{ lb})$; $x = 2,255$ mg.

36. d. Setup: $(220 \text{ mg})/(5 \text{ ml}) = (x \text{ mg})/(473 \text{ ml})$; $x = 20,812$ mg, but we want grams—so convert to grams; $x = 20.81$ g.

37. b. Setup: $(220 \text{ mg})/(5 \text{ ml}) = (120 \text{ mg})/(x \text{ ml})$; $x = 2.7$ ml.

38. c. $(2.7 \text{ ml})(2)(120) = 648$ ml needed; 648 ml – 473 ml = 175 ml short, which comes to 32 days short.

39. a. Setup: $(3 \text{ ml paregoric})/(15 \text{ ml solution}) = (x \text{ ml paregoric})/(5 \text{ ml})$; $x = 1$ ml.

40. d. Setup: $(\$3.45)/(15 \text{ g}) = (x)/(120 \text{ g})$; $x = \$27.60$.

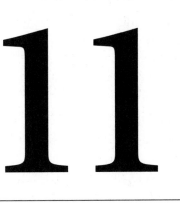

11 ▶ Pharmacy Math III

CHAPTER OVERVIEW

The last two chapters allowed us to review basic mathematics and different systems of measurement, as well as use the method of ratio and proportion to solve both concentration and conversion problems commonly seen in the pharmacy setting. This chapter will include these concepts, as well as introduce problem solving using percents. This chapter will also cover other aspects of problem solving found on the national exam: dosage calculations, the pricing of prescriptions in the retail setting, temperature conversions, etc.

KEY TERMS	
allegation	dosage
AWP	Fahrenheit
Celsius	flow rate
concentration	markup
cost	ratio strength
dilution	stock solution

Learning to calculate **dosages** correctly is an extremely important skill—especially when calculating doses for prescription and medication orders, as well as the correct volume of IV admixtures to add to an IV solution.

Sometimes a technician will receive a prescription or chart order for a dosage of drug that differs from a drug's usual form or what the pharmacy has in stock. In this scenario, the pharmacy technician will have to calculate a correct dose of drug. Although all calculation type problem solving should be checked by a pharmacist before a dose reaches the patient, it is important that the pharmacy technician understand how to perform the necessary calculations. The use of a calculator is always necessary in performing calculations, but you must still have basic math skills to set up problems and to use the calculator correctly.

Understanding Medication Labels

Every medication has a label containing essential information. When filling a prescription or chart order, to reduce the risk of a medication error, always check the medication label in the following three instances:

1. when removing the medication from stock
2. when preparing the dose for dispensing
3. when returning the stock bottle to inventory or discarding the empty container

Most oral medications dispensed in a retail setting are supplied in bulk containers, while most oral medications given in the hospital setting are available in packages containing single (unit) doses.

Some medications may actually be a combination of two or more drugs into one dosage form. These drugs are usually prescribed by the number of capsules, tablets, or milliliters, or by the brand name rather than by dosage strength. For example, the drug Augmentin® suspension contains the mixed ratio of 250 mg of amoxicillin and 62.5 mg of clavulanate potassium per 5 mL.

Tablets and capsules are supplied in the dosage most frequently used. Many tablets and capsules are supplied in multiple strengths. Some doses may require two or more dosage forms for the proper dose. Some tablets may be scored, which means they are marked so they can be divided in half or quarters to achieve the correct dose. It is safest and most accurate to give the fewest number of whole, undivided tablets as possible. Enteric-coated tablets or sustained-release capsules should not be divided or crushed.

Equipment Used in Measuring Doses

If the dose of the medication is a tablet or capsule, there is no special equipment required to measure the dose. However, if the oral dose is a liquid, a dropper may be used for smaller volumes. A specially marked cup, spoon, or oral syringe may be used for larger volumes. If the oral dose is to be administered by dropper, the dropper is usually included in the medication package and is specifically calibrated for that drug. Droppers vary in size and should not be used for any other medication other than the one with which they are dispensed. For safety reasons, oral syringes have a special tip that is different from a syringe used for an injection; a needle cannot be fitted to this type of syringe.

When dosages are supplied or prepared for administration by parenteral (intravenous, intramuscular, or subcutaneous) injections, there are a variety of sizes of syringes used. Most syringes are calibrated in milliliters. But an insulin syringe is specially calibrated to measure and administer insulin in units instead of milliliters. Typically, a U-100 syringe is used, which means there are 100 units of insulin per milliliter. U-100 syringes are available in 50 or 100 unit sizes. When using an insulin syringe, always make sure the **concentration** on the syringe matches the concentration on the insulin vial. Some syringes are prefilled by the manufacturer with a single dose of drug that is ready for use. When a nurse needs to administer less than the pre-filled dose, he or she simply discards the extra medication before giving it to the patient.

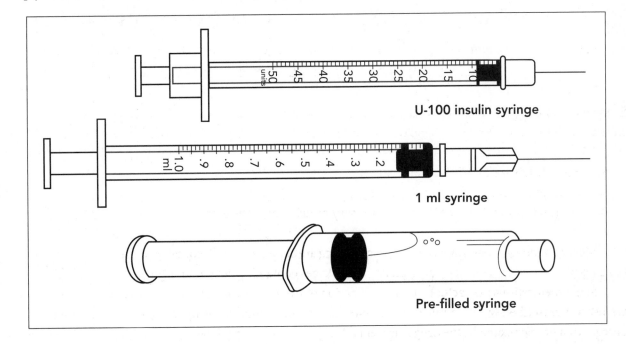

U-100 insulin syringe

1 ml syringe

Pre-filled syringe

Calculating Doses

In practice, it is often necessary to calculate an ordered dose to be composed from various doses or strengths that you have on hand. For example, a physician may order a drug dose that is one and one-half times the strength of the tablet that is available commercially. In this simple example, it would be clear that the dose would be one and one-half tablets. A more complex example is a pediatric dose that you would have to calculate based on the strength of an available oral suspension. An example would be a liquid formulation of a drug such as Amoxil® with the concentration of 500 mg/5 mL, of which you are asked to give a 120 mg dose.

Oral Dosage Calculations

Healthcare providers prefer oral medication dosages because they are convenient for the patient to take, do not require that the skin is punctured for administration, and are usually more economical because the production cost is lower than for other dosage forms.

Sometimes the prescriber's order is written in one system of measurement and the drug is supplied in another. If that is the case, it will be necessary for you to convert one of the measurements so that they are both in either the apothecary or metric systems.

Example: The doctor's order is written: "Lopressor® 100 mg by mouth bid." The drug container is labeled: "Lopressor® 50 mg per tablet." What is the dose the patient should take?

Although common sense may tell you what the answer would be, you can also use ratio and proportion to easily find how many tablets you need to use.

Set up the proportion: have = want

1 tablet/50 mg = x tablets/100 mg

Cross multiply to get this equation: (1 tablet) (100 mg) = (x tablets) (50 mg)

Solve for x by dividing both sides by 50 mg: x tablets = (1 tablet) (100 mg)/50 mg = 2 tablets

So the patient should be taking two tablets by mouth twice a day.

Let's try another one:

Example: "Ampicillin 0.5 g po qid" is prescribed. The dose available is 250 mg/capsule. How many capsules should the RN give the patient?

Set up the proportion: have = want

1 capsule/250 mg = x capsules/0.5 g

In this setup, our units do *not* match in the denominator. In this case, we would need to do a conversion to either change grams to milligrams or milligrams to grams to make them match. Let's change 0.5 g to milligrams:

Set up the proportion: 1 g/1,000 mg = 0.5 g/x mg

What you have in common from your list of ten conversions is what you "have."

Cross multiply to get this equation: (1 g) (x mg) = (0.5 g) (1,000 mg)

Solve for x by dividing both sides by 1 g: x mg = (0.5 g) (1,000 mg)/1 g = 500 mg

Now we can begin anew with our units matching in both the numerator and the denominator of our proportion.

Set up the proportion: have = want

1 capsule/250 mg = x capsules/500 mg

Cross multiply to get this equation: (1 capsule) (500 mg) = (x capsules) (250 mg)

Solve for x by dividing both sides by 250 mg: x capsules = (1 capsule) (500 mg)/250 mg = 2 capsules

So the nurse would give two capsules by mouth four times a day.

Let's try another one:

Example: The order reads, "Codeine gr ss po q4h." The drug label states "Codeine Sulfate 30 mg." How many tabs are given?

Set up the proportion:

have = want

1 tablet/30 mg = x tablet/gr ss

Again, in this setup our units do *not* match in the denominator. In this case we would need to do a conversion to change milligrams to grains or grains to milligrams to make them match. Let's change grains to milligrams :

Also realize that gr ss is the same as gr $\frac{1}{2}$ or 0.5 gr.

Set up the proportion:

1 gr/60 mg = 0.5 gr/x mg

Cross multiply to get this equation:

(1 gr) (x mg) = (0.5 gr) (60 mg)

Solve for x by dividing both sides by 1 g:

x mg = (0.5 gr) (60 mg)/1 gr = 30 mg

Now we can solve for how many codeine tablets are needed.

Set up the proportion:

1 tablet/30 mg = x tablet/30 mg

Cross multiply to get this equation:

(1 tablet) (30 mg) = (x tablet) (30 mg)

Solve for x by dividing both sides by 30 mg:

x tablet= (1 tablet) (30 mg)/30 mg = 1 tablet

So the nurse would give one tablet by mouth four times a day.

Let's try another one:

Example: The MD orders, "KCl 40 mEq by mouth now." The label on the liquid container reads, "KCl 20 mEq/15 mL." What is the correct dose?

Set up the proportion:

20 mEq/15 mL = 40 mEq/x mL

Cross multiply to get this equation:

(20 mEq) (x mL) = (40 mEq) (15 mL)

Solve for x by dividing both sides by 20 mEq:

x mL = (40 mEq) (15 mL)/(20 mEq) = 30 mL

Parenteral Dosage Calculations

Parenteral means that a drug is administered by means other than through the alimentary (GI) tract (such as by intramuscular or intravenous injection). Drugs are administered parenterally when they cannot be taken by mouth or when more rapid action is desirable. Medications administered parenterally are absorbed directly into the bloodstream. The amount of drug required can be determined more accurately when compounding a parenteral dose. This administration technique is necessary for patients who are unconscious, uncooperative, or have been designated "NP0" (nothing by mouth).

Drugs supplied for parenteral use are available as liquids or powders, packaged in a variety of forms. If the drug is supplied as a powder, it must be reconstituted with a diluent (liquid) and completely dissolved to a specific concentration in order to calculate the correct dose.

Accurate measurements of medications that are to be administered by the parenteral route require the use of a syringe. Syringes come in a variety of sizes, and the size selected to measure the dose depends on the amount and type of medication to be administered.

Example: The drug order reads, "Demerol® 35 mg IM every three to four hours as needed for pain." The pre-filled syringe on hand has a label that reads, "Meperidine HCl 50 mg/mL." What is the correct dose in mL?

Note: Demerol® is the trade name for meperidine HCL.

Set up the proportion: have = want

50 mg/1 mL = 35 mg/x mL

Cross multiply to get this equation: (50 mg) (x mL) = (35 mg) (1 mL)

Solve for x by dividing both sides by 50 mg: x mL = (35 mg) (1 mL)/(50 mg) = 0.7 mL

So the order would be for: Demerol® 0.7 mL IM every three to four hours as needed for pain.

Let's do another one:

Example: The drug order says, "Cleocin® 150 mg IM q12h." This drug is available: "Clindamycin PO$_4$ 300 mg/2 mL." What is the correct dose in mL?

Set up the proportion: have = want

300 mg/2 mL = 150 mg/x mL

Cross multiply to get this equation: (300 mg) (x mL) = (150 mg) (2 mL)

Solve for x by dividing both sides by 300 mg: x mL = (150 mg) (2 mL)/(300 mg) = 1 mL

The dose would be 1 mL IM every 12 hours.

Quantity Calculations

You may be asked to calculate the number of doses, the total amount of drug to be administered, or the size of an individual dose.

Calculating Number of Doses

You may have to calculate the number of doses contained in a specific amount of drug. You do this to determine whether you can prepare a sufficient number of doses with the starting materials at hand or if you must acquire additional drugs before beginning your compounding.

Example: How many 10 mg doses are in 1 g?

Set up the proportion: 1 dose/10 mg = x doses/1 g

As you can see, the units do not match in the denominator, so let's make them match.

Set up the proportion: 1 g/1,000 mg = x g/10 mg

Cross multiply to get this equation: (1 g) (10 mg) = (x g) (1,000 mg)

Solve for x by dividing both sides by 1,000 mg: x g = (1 g) (10 mg)/(1,000 mg) = 0.01 g

New setup: 1 dose/0.01 g = x doses/1 g

Cross multiply to get this equation: (1 dose) (1 g) = (x doses) (0.01 g)

Solve for x by dividing both sides by 0.01 g: x doses = (1 dose) (1 g)/(0.01 g) = 100 doses

Calculating the Total Amount of a Drug

You will frequently have to calculate the total amount of drug to dispense, or the total amount of drug a patient has received, when you know the size of each dose and the number of doses.

Example: FeSo4 220 mg/5 mL, 360 mL

Directions: 200 mg po qd × 40 days

What is the total volume necessary for this medication to last the full 40 days?

First of all, we do not know that the individual dose is 200 mg, so our first step would be to solve for that quantity.

Set up the proportion: 220 mg/5 mL = 200 mg/x mL

Cross multiply to get this equation: (220 mg) (x mL) = (200 mg) (5 mL)

Solve for x by dividing both sides by 220 mg: x mL = (200 mg)(5 mL)/(220 mg) = 4.55 mL

The next step would simply be to use your answer (dose), plug it into the directions, and multiply to get the total exact volume.

Directions: 200 mg by mouth once a day for 40 days

Understand that 200 mg is the same as 4.55 mL.

Directions: (4.55 mL) (1) (40) = 182 mL.

Let's try another one:

Example: How many milliliters of ampicillin 250 mg/5 mL suspension do you have to dispense if the patient needs to take "ii tsp qid × 7d"?

This question may be tricky if you try to use the concentration to solve it, as there is no need to do so. The directions (or more specifically, the dose) are a volume measurement, so you need not know the concentration to solve. In other words, two teaspoonsful is a volume, so you need to find out how many milliliters equal two teaspoonsful, plug this into your directions, and multiply.

Set up the proportion: 1 tsp/5 mL = 2 tsp/x mL

Cross multiply to get this equation: (1 tsp) (x mL) = (2 tsp) (5 mL)

Solve for x by dividing both sides by 1 tsp: x mL = (2 tsp) (5 mL)/(1 tsp) = 10 mL

The next step would be simply to use your answer (dose), plug it into the directions, and multiply to get the total exact volume.

Directions: How many milliliters are needed if the patient needs to take 10 mL four times a day for seven days?

Understand that two teaspoonsful are the same as 10 mL.

Directions: (10 mL) (4) (7) = 280 mL

Weight and Individual Dose Problem Solving

Example: What dose, in milligrams, would you give a patient who weighs 234 lb if the drug literature states the dose should be 0.5 mg/5 mL?

Set up the proportion: have = want

0.5 mg/kg = x mg/234 lb

In this case, what you have and want is given in your problem.

When you create a proportion, the units on top (numerator) on both sides must be equal, as well as the units on bottom (denominator) on both sides. In both numerators we see milligrams, but in the denominators we see kilograms and pounds, so they do not match. You must make them match by converting either pounds to kilograms or kilograms to pounds. We suggest changing kilograms to pounds, as this is one of your ten conversions: 1 kg = 2.2 lb.

New setup: 0.5 mg/2.2 lb = x mg/234 lb

Now the units match and we can go ahead and solve!

Cross multiply to get this equation: (0.5 mg) (234 lb) = (x mg) (2.2 lb)

Solve for x by dividing both sides by 2.2 lb: x mg = (0.5 mg) (234 lb)/(2.2 lb) = 53.19 mg

If we were asked the same problem and given a concentration of drug, we could easily solve how much of the drug to dispense as well.

Example: What dose, in milligrams, would you give a patient who weighs 234 lb if the drug literature states that the dose should be 0.5 mg/5 mL? If we have the drug available in the concentrated strength of 100 mg/5 mL 473 mL, how many milliliters would we give this patient for one dose?

Set up the proportion: 100 mg/5 mL = 53.19 mg/x mL

Cross multiply to get this equation: (100 mg) (x mL) = (53.19 mg) (5 mL)

Solve for x by dividing both sides by 100: x mL = (53.19 mg) (5 mL)/(100) = 2.66 mL

Percent Problem Solving

Percents give us information about the concentration in liquid such as IV solutions, or in topical formulations like ointments and creams. A percent is defined as the amount of active drug in grams per 100 mL or 100 g. The number in front of the percent sign always indicates how much active drug is inside the container and is *always in grams*.

The percent can be defined as a ratio, in the respect it will always be the amount of active drug (in grams) over 100, which would be the volume (mL) or amount of base (g) in a topical formulation.

Example: 5%

This would be defined as 5 g/100 mL if we are talking about a liquid formulation.
This would be defined as 5 g/100 g if we are talking about a topical formulation.

Example: dextrose 5% in water

This would be defined as 5 g dextrose/100 mL water

Example: hydrocortisone 2%

This would be defined as 2 g hydrocortisone powder/100 g base.

When setting up a ratio and proportion type of problem for percents, the rule is always to define the percent as information you "have."

Example: How many grams of dextrose 5% in water are in a 500 mL IV bag?

Setup:
$$\text{have} = \text{want}$$
$$5\text{ g}/100\text{ mL} = x\text{ g}/500\text{ mL}$$

For percents, what you have is simply the definition of your percent.

Cross multiply to get this equation:
$$(5\text{ g})\,(500\text{ mL}) = (x\text{ g})\,(100\text{ mL})$$

Solve for x by dividing both sides by 100 mL:
$$x\text{ g} = (5\text{ g})\,(500\text{ mL})/(100\text{ mL}) = 25\text{ g}$$

Let's try another one:

Example: How many grams of NaCl are in 0.9% NaCl 1,000 mL? (Note: NaCL is sodium chloride.)

Setup:
$$0.9\text{ g}/100\text{ mL} = x\text{ g}/1{,}000\text{ mL}$$

Cross multiply to get this equation:
$$(0.9\text{ g})\,(1{,}000\text{ mL}) = (x\text{ g})\,(100\text{ mL})$$

Solve for x by dividing both sides by 100 mL:
$$x\text{ g} = (0.9\text{ g})\,(1{,}000\text{ mL})/(100\text{ mL}) = 9\text{ g}$$

When we are talking about IV solutions, we need to understand the abbreviations of the most common IVs as well:

IV SOLUTION	ABBREVIATION	WHAT IS IN IT
dextrose 5% water	D5W	5 g dextrose in 100 mL sterile water
0.9% NaCl	normal saline (NS)	0.9 g NaCl in 100 mL sterile water
0.45% NaCl	$\frac{1}{2}$ NS	0.45 g NaCl in 100 mL sterile water
0.22% NaCl	$\frac{1}{4}$ NS	0.225 g NaCl in 100 mL sterile water
D5%/0.9% NaCl	D5NS	5 g dextrose and 0.9% NaCl in 100 mL sterile water
D5%/0.45% NaCl	D5 $\frac{1}{2}$ NS	5 g dextrose and 0.45% NaCl in 100 mL sterile water

Example: How many grams of NaCl are in 1 L of $\frac{1}{2}$ NS?

First, note that $\frac{1}{2}$ NS has a concentration of 0.45% NaCl in water, as indicated in the table above. This is the same as 0.45 g NaCl in 100 mL of water.

Setup: have = want

0.45 g/100 mL = x g/1 L

When you create a proportion, the units on top (numerator) on both sides must be equal as well as the units on bottom (denominator) on both sides. In the numerator we see g in both numerators, but in the denominators we see mL and L, so they do not match. You must make them match by converting either mL to L or L to mL so they will match. We would normally have to set up a conversion proportion to make them match, but in this case we know 1 L is equal to 1,000 mL because that is one of our memorized conversions.

New setup: have = want

0.45 g/100 mL = x g/1,000 mL

Cross multiply to get this equation: (0.45 g) (1,000 mL) = (x g) (100 mL)

Solve for x by dividing both sides by 100 mL: x g = (0.45 g) (1,000 mL)/(100 mL) = 4.5 g

Concentration Expressed As Ratio Strength

Frequently, you will express concentrations of weak solutions as **ratio strength**. For example, epinephrine is available in three concentrations: 1:1,000 (read: one-to-one thousand); 1:10,000; and 1:200. A concentration of 1:1,000 means that there is 1 gm of epinephrine in 1,000 mL of solution. You can use ratio strength to set up the ratios needed to solve problems. For example, 1:200 means the same as 1 g of drug/200 mL of final solution, and 1:10,000 means the same as 1 g of drug/10,000 mL of final solution.

Example: How many milligrams of $KMnO_4$ should you use to prepare 500 mL of a 1:2,500 solution?

A 1:2,500 solution has a concentration of 1 g in 2,500 mL of water.

Setup:
$$\text{have} = \text{want}$$
$$1 \text{ g}/2{,}500 \text{ mL} = x \text{ mg}/500 \text{ mL}$$

In this case, the ratio indicates what you "have."

Again, make sure your units match in both numerators and in both denominators. In this case, we know that 1 g = 1,000 mg.

New setup:
$$1{,}000 \text{ mg}/2{,}500 \text{ mL} = x \text{ mg}/500 \text{ mL}$$

Cross multiply to get this equation:
$$(1{,}000 \text{ mg}) (500 \text{ mL}) = (x \text{ mg}) (2{,}500 \text{ mL})$$

Solve for x by dividing both sides by 2,500 mL:
$$x \text{ mg} = (1{,}000 \text{ mg}) (500 \text{ mL})/(2{,}500 \text{ mL}) = 200 \text{ mg}$$

Dilutions Made from Stock Solutions

Stock solutions are concentrated solutions used to prepare various **dilutions** (less concentrated solutions) of the original stock solution. To prepare a solution of a desired concentration, you must calculate the quantity of stock solution that you must mix with diluent (usually sterile water) to prepare the final product.

As in many problems, there are different ways to solve this. Because we have focused on ratio and proportion, we will use this method to solve this type of problem as well.

Example: You have 10% NaCl stock solution available. You need to prepare 200 mL of 0.5% NaCl solution. How many milliliters of stock solution will you need?

Realize that this question could have easily been written as: You have 10:100 NaCl stock solution available. You need to prepare 200 mL of 0.5:100 NaCl solution. How many milliliters of stock solution will you need?

Step 1: Figure out how many grams are needed to make the final product.

Setup:
$$0.5 \text{ g}/100 \text{ mL} = x \text{ g}/200 \text{ mL}$$

Cross multiply to get this equation:
$$(0.5 \text{ g})(200 \text{ mL}) = (x \text{ g}) (100 \text{ mL})$$

Solve for x by dividing both sides by 100 mL:
$$x \text{ g} = (0.5 \text{ g})(200 \text{ mL})/(100 \text{ mL}) = 1 \text{ g}$$

Understand that it will take 1 g of NaCL to produce the product. Create a proportion to see how many milliliters are needed to produce 1 g.

Step 2:

Setup: 10 g/100 mL = 1 g/x mL

Cross multiply to get this equation: (10 g)(x mL) = (1 g) (100 mL)

Solve for x by dividing both sides by 10 g: x mL = (1 g) (100 mL)/(10 g) = 10 mL

Allegation Problem Solving

If the desired percentage concentration of a solution, ointment, or cream you need for filling a prescription or medication order is not available, you can compound it by mixing stronger and weaker components of the same medication to obtain the desired strength. We refer to this method as **allegation** (also known as the "allegation alternate" method) and use it to determine the number of parts or proportions of each component needed to prepare the specific strength of the final product.

An allegation is set up using a diagram similar to the familiar tic-tac-toe grid in the following manner:

PERCENTAGE		PARTS
the percent concentration of the more concentrated solution (a)		parts of higher concentration needed (d)
	(c)	
the percent concentration of the less concentrated solution* (b)		parts of lower concentration needed (e)
		sum of total parts (f)

*When diluting with water, the percent concentration is always zero.

Step 1: Set up the allegation diagram with the higher percentage in the upper left corner, the lower percentage in the lower left corner, and the desired percentage in the middle.

Step 2: Find the lower right corner by calculating the difference between the more concentrated and the desired concentration; this value represents the number of parts of the lower concentration component: (a – c) = (e).

Derive the upper right corner by calculating the difference between the less concentration and the desired concentration; this value represents the number of parts of the higher concentration component: (b – c) = (d).

The sum of these two numbers is the total number of parts: (d) + (e) = (f).

Step 3: Once you have determined the proportional parts, you may calculate the quantities of the higher and lower strength preparations by the method of ratios.

Quantity of MORE concentrated solution:

(# parts higher/# total parts) (total volume needed to make) = total quantity needed

((d)/(f)) times (total volume needed to make) = total quantity needed

Quantity of LESS concentrated solution:

(# parts lower/# total parts) (total volume needed to make) = total quantity needed

((e)/(f)) times (total volume needed to make) = total quantity needed

Example: You need to make 450 mL of 70% ethyl alcohol, but you have only 95% and 50% ethyl alcohol. What quantities of 95% and 50% ethyl alcohol will you mix to make the final product?

First, set up the allegation diagram:

PERCENTAGE			PARTS
95			20 parts (d)
	70		
50			25 parts (e)
			45 total parts (f)

Quantity of MORE concentrated solution (95%):

((d)/(f)) times (total volume needed to make) = total quantity needed

(20)/(45) (450 mL) = 200 mL

Quantity of LESS concentrated solution (50%):

((e)/(f)) times (total volume needed to make) = total quantity needed

(25)/(45) (450 mL) = 250 mL

Example: You have a 50% solution of isopropyl alcohol and a container of distilled water. What quantities of each of these will you mix to make the final product that is 1,000 mL of a 10% solution?

First, set up the allegation diagram:

PERCENTAGE		PARTS
50		10 parts (d)
	10	
0		40 parts (e)
		50 total parts (f)

Quantity of MORE concentrated solution (50% isopropyl alcohol):

((d)/(f)) times (total volume needed to make) = total quantity needed

(10)/(50) (1,000 mL) = 200 mL

Quantity of LESS concentrated solution (distilled water):

((e)/(f)) times (total volume needed to make) = total quantity needed

(40)/(50) (1,000 mL) = 800 mL

Percent Concentration Problem Solving

Typically, you may be given an amount of active drug over a given volume and asked what percent of the concentration the active drug would be. This can be done easily in one step, unless there are conversions that need to be done.

Example: What percent concentration would 2.4 g/240 mL be?

Set up the proportion: have = want

2.4 g/240 mL = x g/100 mL

As with previous question types, always put what you are given as information you "have." For information you want, that is your definition of a percent, which is always: x g/100 mL or g.

Cross multiply to get this equation: (2.4 g) (100 mL) = (x g) (240 mL)

Solve for x by dividing both sides by 240 mL: x g = (2.4 g) (100 mL)/(240 mL) = 1 g

Note: 1 g/100 mL is 1%.

IV Flow Rate, Dosage, and Infusion Time Calculations

IV fluid orders indicate the amount of an IV fluid to be administered to a patient and the length of time over which it is to be given. Before a nurse can administer an IV, he or she must know the **flow rate** for the intravenous solution. Using flow rates, you can calculate the volume of fluid and/or the amount of drug a patient will be receiving over a certain time. Alternatively, if you know the volume of fluid infused and the duration of the infusion, you can calculate the flow rate in mL/min or gtts/min.

Calculating Flow Rate Using Ratio and Proportion

Example: D5W 1,000 mL is to run over eight hours. For how many milliliters per minute would you set your administration pump?

Setup: have = want

In the setup what you have is given, as well as what you want.

$$1,000 \text{ mL}/8 \text{ hours} = x \text{ mL}/1 \text{ min}$$

When you create a proportion, the units on top (numerator) on both sides must be equal as well as the units on bottom (denominator) on both sides. In the denominator we see hours and minutes. Convert hours to minutes so they match. Conversion needed: one hour = 60 minutes, then eight hours = 480 minutes.

New setup: $1,000 \text{ mL}/480 \text{ min} = x \text{ mL}/1 \text{ min}$

Now the units match and we can go ahead and solve!

Cross multiply to get this equation: $(1,000 \text{ mL}) (1 \text{ min}) = (x \text{ mL}) (480 \text{ min})$

Solve for x by dividing both sides by 480 min: $x \text{ mL/min} = (1,000 \text{ mL}) (1 \text{ min})/(480 \text{ min}) = 2.08 \text{ mL/min}$

If you are ever asked for drops (gtts) per minute, you will always be given a drop factor, because different solutions have different densities or weights which will cause the amount of drops per mL of a particular solution to be different. A drop factor is the amount of drops per the volume of 1 mL of that particular solution. In the previous example problem, let's say they wanted to know gtts/min if the drop factor was 12 gtts/1 mL.

Step 1: Determine milliliters per minute as you did before, where you found the answer to be 2.08 mL/min. Multiply this by the drop factor given to get the drops per minute.

Step 2: (2.08 mL) (12 gtts) = 14.08 gtts/min

Other Types of Problem Solving

There may be other types of problem solving on the exam that do not require the use of ratio and proportion. Most of these will require basic math skills in addition, subtraction, multiplication, or division.

Retail Calculations

In order to practice in a retail pharmacy setting, you must be familiar with terms associated with retail calculations.

Cost refers to the amount of money that the pharmacy spent to acquire the item. This amount is the basis for calculations done in a retail setting. Obviously, pharmacists cannot sell an item for the same amount that they paid for it; they would quickly go bankrupt. Since you must show a profit to stay in business, some kind of increase in selling price is necessary.

Markup is the difference between the cost of an item and the price for which the item sells. The markup varies from establishment to establishment and depends on a number of factors, such as cost of goods, utilities, salaries of employees, consumables used in normal business activities, and the amount of profit desired. Markups are generally given in percents, but realize that sometimes you may see a markdown as well!

A dispensing fee is what the pharmacy charges the customer for filling the prescription.

Selling price is the actual dollar amount the customer pays for the product or service.

> selling price = (cost) (+ markup or – markdown) + (dispensing fee)

Example: You are to dispense 30 tablets that cost the pharmacy $56.00 with a 10% markup and a $6.00 dispensing fee. How much are you going to charge the patient?

> selling price = ($56.00) + (10% markup) + ($6.00)

To find markup price: Using your calculator, first find out what a 10% markup is for a $56.00 cost. Simply enter 56.00 and multiply this by .10, then hit the enter key. This will give you your markup, which is $5.60.

> new selling price = ($56.00)+ ($5.60) + ($6.00) = $67.60

Let's try another one:

Example: You are to dispense 100 tablets. The cost for 1,000 of the tabs is $345.00, with a markup of 12% and a dispensing fee of $12.00. How much are you going to charge this patient?

In this case, we need to find out the cost of 100 tablets.

Setup: (1,000 tablets)/($345.00) = (100 tablets)/(x)

Cross multiply to get this equation: (1,000 tablets)(x) = (100 tablets)($345.00)

Solve for x by dividing both sides by 1,000 tablets: x = $34.50

Now we can solve our pricing problem:

> selling price = (cost) + (markup or – markdown) + (dispensing fee)
>
> new selling price = ($34.50) + ($4.14) + ($12.00) = $50.64

Pricing can also include the **average wholesale price (AWP)**, which is the price for the drug if the pharmacy is billing an insurance company (known as third-party billing). In this case, the customer would have a co-payment as well, and we would deduct this co-payment when billing the insurance company, as the customer has already paid this to us.

selling price = (AWP) + (markup or – markdown) + (dispensing fee) – (co-payment)

Example: A customer comes into the pharmacy with insurance and pays a co-payment of $10.00. The pharmacy needs to bill the insurance company for 60 tablets, of which the AWP is $84.00 with an 8% markup and a $12.00 dispensing fee. For how much will the insurance company be billed?

selling price = (AWP) + (markup or – markdown) + (dispensing fee) – (co-payment)

selling price = ($84.00) + ($6.72) + ($12.00) – ($10.00) = $112.72

Temperature Conversion

Temperature is always measured in the number of degrees centigrade (°C), also known as degrees **Celsius**, or the number of degrees **Fahrenheit** (°F). The Fahrenheit scale establishes the freezing point of water at 32°F and the boiling point at 212°F. The Celsius scale establishes the freezing point of water at 0°C and the boiling point at 100°C.

The differences between the size of the degrees and the freezing points of water determine the values in the conversion formulas.

To convert a given Fahrenheit temperature to Celsius, first subtract 32 and then divide the result by 1.8. The formula is °C = (°F – 32)/1.8.

Example: Convert 98.6°F to °C.

°C = (°F – 32)/1.8

°C = (°98.6 – 32)/1.8

°C = 66.6/1.8

°C = 37

To convert Celsius temperature to Fahrenheit, multiply by 1.8 and add 32. The formula is:

°F = 1.8 × °C + 32°

Example: Convert 35°C to °F.

°F = (1.8 × °C) + 32°

°F = (1.8 × 35°) + 32°

°F = (1.8 × 35°) + 32°

°F = (63°) + 32°

°F = 95°

In pharmacy, we use the Celsius unit of measurement. Refrigerated items should be 2–5 degrees Celsius. Room temperature should be 25–35 degrees Celsius.

Practice Questions

1. When selecting a medication to fill a prescription, you should always read the label
   a. when removing the medication from stock.
   b. when preparing the dose for dispensing.
   c. when returning the stock bottle to inventory or discarding the empty container.
   d. all of the above

2. Most oral medications dispensed in a retail setting are supplied in
   a. unit dose packages.
   b. packages containing a single dose.
   c. liquid form.
   d. bulk containers.

3. The most common dosage forms supplied are
   a. tablets and capsules.
   b. tablets and solutions.
   c. tablets and suppositories.
   d. tablets and suspensions.

4. Which of the following is false regarding droppers?
   a. They are usually included in the drug package.
   b. They may be used for medications other than the ones with which they are packaged.
   c. Droppers included with drug packages are specially calibrated.
   d. They should be used only as directed.

5. Which of the following statements is false?
   a. Tablets and capsules are used mostly due to ease of administration.
   b. Liquid formulation dosing can be exact by using ratio and proportion.
   c. All tablets or capsules can be chewed.
   d. Calculations are an important aspect of what you do in the pharmacy setting.

6. Which of the following statements concerning the administration of insulin is true?
   a. Insulin only comes in a 1 mL syringe.
   b. An insulin syringe is calibrated in milliliters.
   c. The standard for insulin injection would be 1 mL = 100 units of insulin.
   d. The standard for insulin injection would be 1 mL = 50 units of insulin.

7. How much lidocaine is required to prepare 30 mL of a 1:1,000 solution?
   a. 10 mg
   b. 0.03 mg
   c. 30 mg
   d. 300 mg

8. A patient comes in to pay for his or her medication. The cost of the drug is $24.98 with a 7% markup and a $6.00 dispensing fee. How much should the patient be charged?
   a. $24.68
   b. $29.51
   c. $32.73
   d. $38.40

9. 98.6°C is what temperature Fahrenheit?
   a. 37°F
   b. 69°F
   c. 177.4°F
   d. 208.4°F

10. If a prescription reads, "Augmentin® 875 mg po bid × 10 days," how many milliliters of Augmentin® 250 mg per 5 mL are required to fill a ten-day supply?
    a. 5 mL
    b. 17.5 mL
    c. 35 mL
    d. 350 mL

11. If 250 mg of cefazolin powder are diluted with water to 50 mL, what is the percent concentration of drug in the final solution?
    a. 10%
    b. 5%
    c. 1%
    d. 0.5%

12. How much erythromycin is in 60 mL of topical erythromycin 2% solution?
    a. 2 g
    b. 2.4 g
    c. 0.6 g
    d. 1.2 g

13. How many 500 mg capsules of doxycycline are required to prepare 250 mL of 2% solution?
    a. 3
    b. 5
    c. 6
    d. 10

14. If three 150 mg capsules of clindamycin are added to 150 mL of 1% Cleocin® topical solution, what is the final percent of clindamycin in the mixture?
    a. 1.5%
    b. 1.3%
    c. 1.1%
    d. 0.9%

15. If an adult dose is 5 mg/kg body weight. What dose would we give a 123 lb adult?
    a. 71.42 mg
    b. 184.5 mg
    c. 224.5 mg
    d. 307.5 mg

16. How many grams of sodium chloride are required to make 750 mL of normal saline?
    a. 1.35 g
    b. 2.50 g
    c. 6.75 g
    d. 12.25 g

17. How much of a 1:1,000 stock solution is needed to make 240 mL 1:3,000 solution?
    a. 40 mL
    b. 60 mL
    c. 80 mL
    d. 100 mL

18. 101.8°F is what temperature in degrees centigrade?
    a. 24.56°C
    b. 38.77°C
    c. 39°C
    d. 215.24°C

19. The prescription is written as "metoprolol 100 mg by mouth twice a day." The drug container is labeled, "metoprolol 50 mg per tablet." What dose should the patient take?
    a. one tablet once a day
    b. two tablets once a day
    c. one tablet twice a day
    d. two tablets twice a day

20. A prescription is for ampicillin 0.5 g by mouth four times a day. The available dose is 250 mg per capsule. How many capsules should the nurse give the patient each day?
    a. 1
    b. 2
    c. 4
    d. 8

21. The order reads, "morphine gr ss po every four hours as needed for pain." The drug label states, "morphine sulfate 30 mg." How many tablets should be given for each dose?
    a. 1
    b. 2
    c. 3
    d. 4

22. The physician orders, "KCl 60 mEq by mouth now." The label on the package reads, "KCl 20 mEq per 15 mL." What is the correct dose?
    a. 15 mL
    b. 30 mL
    c. 45 mL
    d. 60 mL

23. The drug order is for "morphine sulfate 15 mg IV." Morphine is available as 4 mg per milliliter. What is the correct dose, in milliliters?
    a. 1.25 mL
    b. 2.5 mL
    c. 3.75 mL
    d. 5 mL

24. If 500 mL of Fortaz® solution containing 2 g of drug should be administered via slow IV infusion over six hours, what is the rate of infusion?
    a. 25 mL/hr
    b. 83.33 mL/hr
    c. 167.67 mL/hr
    d. 333.33 mL/hr

25. How many 20 mg doses are in 1 g?
    a. 10
    b. 25
    c. 50
    d. 100

26. How many milliliters of amoxicillin suspension do you dispense if the patient needs to take two teaspoonsful four times a day for ten days?
    a. 140
    b. 200
    c. 280
    d. 400

27. How many 50 mg tablets of drug A are needed to make a 1:400 500 mL liquid formulation?
    a. 10 tablets
    b. 20 tablets
    c. 25 tabs
    d. 35 tablets

28. You have 10% sodium chloride stock solution available. You need to prepare 300 mL of 3% sodium chloride solution. How many milliliters of stock solution will you use?
    a. 45 mL
    b. 90 mL
    c. 135 mL
    d. 180 mL

29. Robitussin DM® contains 15 mg of dextro-methorphan in a teaspoon of solution. How many grams of drug are present in a pint container (480 mL)?
    a. 0.45 g
    b. 1.44 g
    c. 0.015 g
    d. 2.45 g

30. A patient is to receive a total of 120 mg of furo-semide each day and takes one dose every six hours. How many milligrams are in each dose?
    a. 10
    b. 20
    c. 30
    d. 40

31. A patient who weighs 50 kg is to receive acyclovir every eight hours. The recommended dose is 15 mg/kg/d. What is the individual dose for this patient?

a. 125 mg

b. 250 mg

c. 500 mg

d. 1,000 mg

32. How much of a D10W and sterile water for injection are needed to prepare a D8W 250 mL?

a. 200 mL D10W/50 mL sterile water

b. 50 mL D10W/200 mL sterile water

c. 150 mL D10W/100 mL sterile water

d. 100 mL D10W/150 mL sterile water

33. How much 70% alcohol is required to prepare 750 mL of 20% alcohol?

a. 501.01 mL

b. 335.16 mL

c. 214.28 mL

d. 428.12 mL

34. In what proportion should 3% acetic acid and 1% acetic acid be mixed to prepare 200 mL of 2.5% acetic acid?

a. 150 and 50 mL

b. 100 and 100 mL

c. 75 and 125 mL

d. 175 and 25 mL

35. You are billing an insurance company for the following medication:

Drug A: 60 tabs with an AWP of $590.00 for 1,000 tablets with a 6% markdown, a $5.00 dispensing fee, and a co-payment of $10.00

How much should be billed to the insurance company?

a. $28.28

b. $32.14

c. $41.80

d. $61.30

36. How many milliliters of purified water should be added to 45% alcohol to prepare 750 mL of 25% alcohol?

a. 125 mL

b. 222 mL

c. 333.33 mL

d. 451 mL

Use the following information to solve problem 37 and 38.

- 0.45% NaCl 500 mL
- infuse over six hours
- drop factor: 12 gtts/mL

37. How many gtts/min would you set the administration pump for this IV?

a. 12

b. 13

c. 17

d. 21

38. How many milligrams of NaCl are in this IV?

a. 2,250

b. 4,500

c. 9,000

d. 12,000

39. 20 mL of 10% KCl solution, 50 mL of 25% NaHCO3 solution, and 30 mL of 20% CaCl2 solution are mixed with 1,000 mL of D5W. The infusion should be administered over eight hours. What is the flow rate?

  a. 79.14 mL/h

  b. 84.3 mL/h

  c. 108.06 mL/h

  d. 137.5 mL/h

40. The most common system of measure used in the pharmacy setting is

  a. the apothecary system of measurement.

  b. the gothic system of measurement.

  c. the household system of measurement.

  d. the metric system of measurement.

Answers and Explanations

1. d. You should always read the label three times when filling a prescription or compounding a sterile product: once when you select the product, once when filling the order, and once when returning the drug to stock or discarding the empty container.

2. d. Unit dose packages and packages containing a single dose are more common in hospitals, and liquids are not dispensed as frequently as tablets or capsules.

3. a. The most common dosage forms supplied are tablets and capsules.

4. b. Droppers are calibrated for the solution with which they are packaged. Using them with a different product may result in a dosage error.

5. c. Not all tablets or capsules can be chewed, crushed, or cut, as some are long-acting or formulated for a sustained release. By doing so, the patient would get the full strength of the medication at once.

6. c. Standard insulin is 1 mL = 100 units. This makes solving insulin problems easy, as long as you know this information (which they will not tell you on the national exam). Example: How many milliliters equal 35 units of insulin? (1 mL)/(100 units) = (x mL)/(35 units); x = 0.35 mL.

7. c. A 1:1,000 solution contains 1 g in 1,000 mL of solution, which is 1 mg/mL. So 30 mg would be needed to prepare 30 mL of lidocaine solution. 1,000 mg/1,000 mL = 30 mg/x mL.

8. c. The cost of a drug is 24.98 with a 7% markup and a $6.00 dispensing fee. Selling price = cost + 7% markup + $6.00; $24.98 + $1.75 + $6.00 = $32.73.

9. d. 98.6°C is what temperature Fahrenheit? F = (32) + (1.8) (C degrees) = 208.4 degrees F.

10. d. Setup: (250 mg)/(5 mL) = (875 mg)/(x mL) will give you the individual dose of 1.43 mL. Then plug the individual dose in your directions and multiply: (17.5 mL)(2)(10) = 350 mL.

11. d. Setup: (0.25 g)/(50 mL) = (x g)/(100 mL); x = 0.5 g; 0.5 g/100 mL is the definition of 0.5%.

12. d. A 2% solution contains (2 g/100 mL). Setup: (2 g/100 mL) = (x g/60 mL); x = 1.2 g.

13. d. A 2% solution contains (2 g/100 mL). Setup: (2 g/100 mL) = (x g/250 mL); x = 5 g; new setup: (1 capsule/500 mg) = (x capsules/5,000 mg); x = 10 capsules.

14. b. A 1% solution contains 1 g/100 mL, so 150 mL of a 1% solution would contain 1.5 g. Three capsules each containing 150 mg contain a total of 450 mg, or 0.45 g. This 0.45 g is added to the 1.5 g already present in the 150 mL for a final concentration of 1.95 g/150 mL. This equals a concentration of 1.3% (1.3 g/100 mL).

15. d. Remember that 1 kg = 2.2 lb; (5 mg/2.2 lb) = (x mg/123 lb); x = 307.5 g.

16. c. Normal saline is 0.9% sodium chloride solution, containing 0.9 g of NaCl per 100 mL. (0.9 g/100 mL) = (x g/750 mL); x = 6.75 g.

17. c. Find out how many grams are in the product, then place that into your stock solution to find out how many milliliters are needed. Setup: (1 g/3,000 mL) = (x g/240 mL); x = 0.08 g. New setup: (1 g/1,000 mL) = (0.08 g/x mL); x = 80 mL.

18. c. C = (5/9)(F − 32); C = (5/9) (101.8 − 32) = 39 degrees Celsius.

19. d. Setup: (1 tab/50 mg) = (x tab/100 mg); x = two tablets.

20. d. Setup: (1 cap/250 mg) = (x cap/500 mg); directions: (2 caps)(4) = 8 caps per day.

21. a. Setup: (gr 1/60 mg) = (gr ss/x mg); gr ss is equal to 30 mg, and the tablet strength is 30 mg, so one tablet is needed per dose.

22. c. Setup: (20 mEq/15 mL) = (60 mEq/x mL); x = 45 mL.

23. c. Setup: (4 mg/1 mL) = (15 mg/x mL); x = 3.75 mL.

24. b. Setup: 500 mL/6 hr = x mL/1 hr; x = 83.33 mL/hr.

25. c. Setup: (20 mg/1 dose) = (1,000 mg/x doses); x = 50 doses.

26. d. Find the individual dose, then plug it into the directions and multiply: 2 tsp = 10 mL. Final setup: (10 mL)(4)(10) = 400 mL .

27. c. Find the total amount of the drug needed. Setup: (1 g/400 mL) = (x g/500 mL); x = 1.25 g. Then find how many tabs are needed: (1 tab/50 mg) = (1,250 mg/x tabs); x = 25 tabs.

28. b. Define 10% as (10 g/100 mL). Find the total amount of grams needed for the product, then insert that answer in your stock solution to find out how many milliliters are needed. Final setup: (10 g/100 mL) = (9 g/x mL) = 90 mL needed.

29. b. Setup: (15 mg/5 mL) = (x mg/480 mL); x = 1,440 mg; then covert to grams for answer.

30. c. Dosing every six hours is four doses per day. 120 mg/day divided by 4 doses/day = 30 mg/dose. Or you can solve using the following setup: (120 mg/4 doses) = (x mg/1 dose).

31. b. Setup for total daily dose: (15 mg/1 kg) = (x mg/50 kg); x = 750 mg. But they are asking for individual daily dose, and there are three doses per day, so: (750 mg/3 doses) = 250 mg.

32. a. Use allegation:

10		8 parts
	8	
0		2 parts

10 total parts
Quantity of higher strength = (8 parts/10 parts) × 250 mL = 200 mL. Quantity of lower strength (water) = (2 parts/10 parts) × 250 mL = 50 mL. Check work by adding the two volumes: 200 mL + 50 mL = 250 mL.

33. c. Use allegation:

70		20 parts
	20	
0		50 parts

70 total parts
Quantity of higher strength = (20 parts/70 parts) × 750 mL = 214.28 mL. Quantity of lower strength (water) = (50 parts/70 parts) × 750 mL = 535.72 mL. Check work by adding the two volumes: 214.28 mL + 535.72 mL = 750 mL.

34. a. Use allegation:

3		5 parts
	5	
1		5 parts

0 total parts
Quantity of higher strength = (1.5 parts/2 parts) × 200 mL = 150 mL. Quantity of lower strength = (0.5 parts/2 parts) × 200 mL = 50 mL. Check work by adding the two volumes: 150 mL + 50 mL = 200 mL.

35. a. Selling price for AWP = (AWP) (+ markup or – markdown) + (dispensing fee) – (co-payment), so ($35.40) – ($2.12) + ($5.00) – ($10.00) = $28.28.

36. c. Use allegation:

45		25 parts
	25	
0		20 parts

45 total parts
Quantity of higher strength = (25 parts/45 parts) × 750 mL = 416.67 mL. Quantity of lower strength = (20 parts/45 parts) × 750 mL = 333.33 mL. Check work by adding the two volumes: 416.67 mL + 333.33 mL = 750 mL.

37. c. Setup: (500 mL/360 min) = (x mL/1 min) = (1.39 mL/1 min). Simply multiply this number by the drop factor: (1.39 mL/1 min)(12 gtts) = 17 gtts/min.

38. a. Setup: (0.45 g/100 mL) = (x g/500 mL); x = 2.25 g, then convert this to milligrams.

39. d. Total volume of the solution = 20 + 50 + 30 + 1,000 mL = 1,100 mL. Setup: (1,100 mL/8 hr) = (x mL/1 hr); x = 137.5 mL/hr.

40. d. The metric system is the most common system of measure used in the pharmacy setting.

12 ▶ Working in the Pharmacy Setting

CHAPTER OVERVIEW

The many common duties performed by a pharmacy technician will be discussed in this chapter. In order to be an effective member of the pharmacy team, it is important for a technician to know what his or her role is in each process performed in the pharmacy. This chapter will begin with the importance of the policy and procedures manual and conclude with different roles required of the pharmacy technician in different settings, including the hospital.

KEY TERMS

additives	drug wholesaler	IV admixture
aminosyn	electrolytes	IV room
ampule	filter needle or straw	intravenous piggy back
cassette	flow rate	laminar flow hood
centralized pharmacy	formulary	lipids
clean room	gauge	luer lock
controlled substances	high efficiency particulate air (HEPA) filters	large volume parenterals
DEA Form 222	home-care setting	medication error
decentralized pharmacy		medication order
direct purchasing	infusion	outpatient prescription
dose	isopropyl alcohol 70%	

KEY TERMS

periodic automatic
replenishment
patient profile
policy
procedure

purchase order
Pyxis®
quality assurance
quality control
reconstitution

repackaged medications
small volume parenterals
unit dose
vials

Pharmacy technicians fulfill many vital functions as part of the pharmacy organization. Their duties include maintaining and announcing changes to policies and procedures manuals. Technicians also keep the pharmacy running efficiently by managing medication orders and prescriptions, patient profiles, inventory and purchasing control systems, and ensuring quality improvement. Any role that does not require an educated judgment decision is open for the pharmacy technician to fill.

The Policies and Procedures Manual

The policies and procedures manual, found in most pharmacy settings, is used to establish requirements, principles, and protocols to ensure safe and effective operations. It is also used to ensure that when situations arise, they are handled consistently each time. Policies and procedures are a record of previous decisions made that define the way the pharmacy will operate. Specifically, a **policy** is a definite course or method of action selected from among alternatives that provide conditions to guide and determine present and future actions.

Policies and **procedures** also contain the required minimum standards for pharmacy professional organizations and accreditation, as determined by regulatory agencies. For example, required policies include the handling of drug/food interactions, drug recalls, **medication errors**, and adverse drug reactions.

The manual also serves as the basis for the training of new staff. During the orientation of a new employee, the policy manual serves as the standard reference for learning a new job. You will probably review the pharmacy policy and procedure manual as one of the first activities upon starting a new job, and refer to it frequently during your first few weeks.

Established policies and procedures also promote safety in the workplace. Documentation of safety measures to protect the workers and the patients or clients is always part of the policy manual. To ensure safe conduct, staff should refer at all times to policy for guidance in their work patterns, rather than following shortcut methods that another employee may recommend.

Policies and procedures are not static documents. Most policy and procedure manuals undergo annual review and revision. Whenever the department or corporate management makes a change in an official requirement, a new or revised policy or procedure is issued that reflects that change. Generally, if there is a question regarding established protocols, it is the policy and procedures manual we look to for guidance.

Interpreting and Receiving Medication Orders and Prescriptions

Interpreting a **medication order**, or prescription, is the core of a pharmacy technician's responsibilities in any practical setting. Interpreting the prescription is also the first step in processing these orders and initiating the filling of a medication. This section will outline what is necessary for processing each medication order in the appropriate manner.

Medication Orders

A-1 a DOCTORS' ORDERS

Remove TOP carbon copy to send to Pharmacy
File most recent sheet of this number on bottom
1. Write firmly, this form has many copies.
2. Affix date and signature to each set of orders.
3. Write orders to change or discontinue a current order on next blank line.
4. Verbal orders must be signed, dated and timed by physician within 24 hours.
5. Medication orders must include the four character (alpha-numeric) prescriber's code.
6. Medication orders for this patient expire as stated in the "Prescribing Medications for Hospitalized Patients" section of the current UIHC Formulary and Handbook.

DRUG AND IV ORDERS ONLY
DRUG ALLERGIES. TO BE COMPLETED BY PRACTITIONER ONLY.
☐ No Known Allergies
☐ Specialty

DATE TIME	DRUG OR I.V. SOLUTION	DOSE	ROUTE	REGIMEN
3-13-10 1300	Digoxin	.25 mg	po	daily
	Furosemide	40 mg	po	daily
3-13-10	Atenolol	50 mg	po	daily
	Triomcinolone cream	0.1%		Apply TID to rash
	Ds 1/2 NS with 20 m EQk	a/L	IV	to run at 125 ml/hr
	Acetaminophen	650 mg	PO	every 4 hours PRN pain
3-15-10 0800	Discontinue			
	Digoxin	.25 mg	PO	daily
	Begin Digoxin	.125 mg	PO	daily

DATE: 3-13-10 PATIENT CARE UNIT: 4JCW
HOSP #: 88-12345-1
NAME: Stacy Smith
BIRTHDATE: 10-1-39
ADDRESS: Anytown, USA 51234
SS#: 123-00-1234

ADMIT to (unit) _____
Date/time _____
OCCUPANCY CATEGORY: (check only one)
Inpatient: Acute _____
Housed Outpatient: Custodial _____
_____ Recovery _____
Staff Attending Physician Name:

DATE/TIME	DIAGNOSTIC, THERAPEUTIC AND DIETARY ORDERS:

Patients in hospitals and residents of licensed healthcare facilities have their medical records collected, collated, and stored in a paper and/or electronic chart. These records are divided into sections for admissions information (address, insurance, advance directives), laboratory tests, radiology reports, physician's progress notes, chart orders, and other pertinent information groupings.

Chart orders in patient charts include all instructions for patient care. Some facilities use single page physician's order forms; others utilize multiple NCR (carbonless copy) pages so that the second and third copies may be sent to various departments. Some facilities scan the original order and electronically transmit a picture to the pharmacy or other departments. Chart orders are usually written by physicians, but other licensed personnel (pharmacists, nurses, respiratory therapists, etc.) may write orders for their

disciplines, as directed by the physician and approved by medical staff protocols and/or any legal statutes. Orders may include medications, treatments, nursing procedures (record intake and output, temperature every four hours, activity level, diet, etc.), and orders for diagnostic procedures (radiology, ultrasound, etc.).

The pharmacy processes chart orders for medications in a similar fashion to **outpatient prescriptions**. The order must contain the name of the medication, strength, route, frequency, and in certain circumstances, indications for use and/or length of therapy. The orders do not need to specify the quantity to be dispensed, however. The duration of therapy for a particular medication is often the length of the patient's stay. Records of chart order prescriptions must be maintained for a three-year period and must be readily accessible to a board of pharmacy inspector.

Handwritten chart orders must be dated and timed, be legible, have the required elements of the order as designated by the medical staff, and be signed by the prescriber. They must not contain any unapproved abbreviations. Orders written by nurses or other healthcare professionals (as with telephone or in-person orders) must be countersigned by a physician within 24–72 hours. Orders written per prior, approved medical staff protocols do not need to be countersigned by the physician, but by the designated licensee (for medications, usually a pharmacist).

Outpatient Prescription

CARDIOVASCULAR ASSOCIATES, PC
(555)555-5555
1234 Main Street, Suite 567
Anytown, USA 12345
Jane Doe, M.D.
John Smith, M.D.

Name: Smith, John
Address: _____ Date: 3/12/10

Lipitor, 10mg

Refill _2_ times.   J Smith   M.D.

Outpatient prescriptions can be generated four ways:

1. Handwritten by the prescriber, on a preprinted prescription form
2. Generated by a computer and communicated to the pharmacy via fax machine
3. Telephoned to the pharmacy by the prescriber or the prescriber's agent
4. Communicated electronically to the pharmacy via e-mail

All handwritten prescriptions usually contain the physician's information as well as patient's name, birth date, date of prescription, medication information, signature of prescriber, and other relevant information that pertains to the patient (indication for use, pregnancy status, diagnosis, etc.). Electronic and computer-generated prescriptions have many advantages over handwritten prescriptions, as they generally contain more pertinent information (which is not necessarily required) and are much easier to read. Computer programs for electronic prescriptions may contain a database of insurance formulary (medications the insurance company will pay for), the standard generic/trade names of drugs as well as other available information, available strengths, and recommended dosing regimens for a specific diagnosis. The programs range from very simple to very complex, integrated programs which may be able to interface with other integrated programs. Usually, the more specialized the physician's practice, the more complex the program.

Traditional prescription pads are usually preprinted with the name, address, phone number, state license number, and Drug Enforcement Administration number of the prescriber. Many have all of the office's or practice's physicians, physicians' assistants (PA), or nurse practitioners (NP) printed on the form. PAs and NPs may only prescribe drugs as designated by their supervising physician. To prescribe **controlled substances**, they also must have a DEA number. Some physicians will use preprinted prescriptions with drugs, such as prenatal vitamins for obstetric patients or antibiotics for pediatric patients. These may or may not have the physician information preprinted or may have just the physician's signature or stamp. For these, it is the pharmacy's obligation to verify the authenticity of the signature of the prescriber and have the prescriber's information on file.

Secure prescription pads are most commonly used for scheduled, controlled substances. However, individual states require that all reimbursable prescriptions must be written on secure prescription pads. This includes prescriptions for Medicare and Medicaid patients and those patients who qualify for both programs simultaneously. Secure prescriptions are very similar to checks, in that they are printed on watermarked, thermographic paper with specific security enhancements. If the prescription is photocopied, the copy will have "VOID" printed across the face. The secure prescription pads and/or paper stock (for a prescriber that generates computer printed prescriptions) must be obtained from a state licensed printer/distributor. The form must also contain checkboxes for the number of **doses** of each drug on the blank, as outlined in state law.

Schedule II controlled substances must be prescribed on a secure prescription blank and are NOT refillable. All secure prescriptions may be initially filled for up to six months after the prescription date. Schedule III, IV, and V controlled substances may be refilled five times in six months, then must be renewed and assigned a new prescription number. Many pharmacies require the pharmacist/intern to verify all faxed prescriptions for controlled substances, whether they are computer-generated or handwritten prior to faxing.

Telephoned prescriptions are acceptable for all drugs other than those in schedule II, with the exception of some drugs under research clinical trial protocols. Usually a designated person from the physician's staff will phone the prescription in to a pharmacist or a pharmacy intern. Refill authorizations for prescriptions may be taken by a technician. Telephoned prescriptions must be put in writing by the pharmacist or intern, including information like the patient name, date, physician, medication, dose, quantity, and directions. The pharmacist/intern must include information about the person transmitting the prescription (name of physician, nurse, assistant) and initial the prescription.

Faxed prescriptions are usually generated by the physician's office computer straight to the pharmacy fax machine. Refill authorizations may appear as computer-generated, or with a handwritten refill notation and the initials of the designated office staff person.

Some pharmacies have a physician's voicemail service on their automated telephone line. Usually this is used by a physician's staff member to call in refill authorizations. However, occasionally a physician or designee will leave a new prescription on the voicemail. The pharmacist or pharmacist intern will record this information, and it is his or her responsibility to verify the accuracy of the prescriber, patient, and prescription information. Many pharmacists will not accept scheduled substance prescriptions recorded on voicemail and will contact the prescriber for verification.

Electronically communicated prescriptions will become more common as physicians and pharmacists begin using computers that have easily integrated systems. This also allows for easy access to patient, prescriber, and pharmacy information.

Receiving the Order

Regardless of setting, the pharmacy staff receives a copy of the physician's order in a variety of ways. They are delivered to the pharmacy in person or via some mechanical method such as fax transmissions or a pneumatic tube (a tube that transports items throughout the hospital setting) from different nursing units. Orders may also be telephoned to the pharmacy. Upon receipt, the order should be reviewed for clarity and completion, then prioritized based upon patient need or physician directives.

Reviewing for Clarity and Completeness

In an inpatient setting, if the pharmacy copy is difficult to read, the original order is in the patient's chart.

Reviewing the original order may clarify it. If any order cannot be read with certainty, the physician must be contacted. Never guess on a medication order. A complete inpatient order will contain patient name, date, drug name, dose, route, and frequency, with the prescriber's signature closing the order. Ideally, the time the order was written and the patient's room number should also appear. In the outpatient setting, the pharmacy staff will have access only to the original prescription. If there is any question regarding any aspect of the prescription, the physician must be contacted for clarification, and a notation must be made regarding the exchange.

Priority of Order

Factors to consider when assigning priority to orders include the time the medication is needed, the seriousness of the condition being treated, and the urgency of other orders waiting to be processed. Prescribers may sometimes indicate the urgency of an order by writing "STAT," "ASAP," or "NOW" on the prescription order. Hospital policy will define the time frame intended by this terminology. Most medication orders do not have an urgency notation from the prescriber and are considered routine orders. The turnaround time for this type of order may be no more than an hour or two, as defined by the hospital pharmacy. Even without a specific urgency notation, orders for code blue (emergency situation) medications, trauma calls, emergency room requests, and medications for patients in surgery should be given top priority. With experience, you will learn which other classes of drugs—such as critical care medications—deserve a higher priority than a routine medication.

Interpreting the Order

Interpreting the order is the most important part of the process because it is the step where most errors occur during the filling process. There are four areas of importance when interpreting an order: identifying the patient, selecting the drug products, dosage, and scheduling medication times. Each area provides a possibility for an error to be made. It is important that each section is entered into the computer carefully to reduce the likelihood of errors.

Identifying the Patient

Compare the patient data on the chart order with the patient data in the computer to make sure they match. In an institutional setting, patient names, unique medical record numbers, room numbers, or account numbers may be used to identify the patient. Once the patient data is brought up on the computer, personal information—such as height, weight, age, and diagnosis—may also appear to ensure the order is correct. Other current medications may appear in the **patient profile**. Before orders are entered into a patient's profile, the profile should be reviewed in relation to the changes indicated on the new orders. The drug should also be checked carefully against the patient's allergy list.

In a retail setting, the patient is identified by the information taken on the prescription and is matched to what is already stored in the database. The most commonly used demographic information includes name, date of birth, and address. Once a patient is identified, the medication information can be entered.

Selecting Drug Products

Prescribers may order by generic or brand name. Selecting drug products requires a working knowledge of both brand and generic names. The dosage form chosen must be compatible with the route of medication delivery (e.g., liquid for nasogastric, or NG, use). In a hospital, consideration must be given as to whether or not the drug order is approved for use in the hospital (on the formulary). The physician may need to be contacted if the drug is not on the formulary. Once a drug is selected, most computer systems will alert the operator if the medication will conflict with preexisting orders or patient's allergies, or if the new medication represents a therapeutic duplication. The pharmacist must be consulted when an alert is posted.

In the retail setting, a medication will be automatically filled as a generic unless otherwise identified by the prescriber. In addition, the dosage form is usually provided on the prescription. After this information is entered, the system will cross-reference the patient's allergies and current medication(s) against the new prescription being filled.

Dosage

The dosage is written in standard units, depending on the drug being prescribed. Units of measure include grams, milligrams, micrograms, milliequivalents, millimoles, units, milliliters, and liters .

Scheduling Medication Times

Medication administration times are often defined by institutional policy or by drug therapy protocol. Such policies may define times for common dosing frequencies or indicate administration time for specific drugs. For example, a "qd" dose will be given daily, often at a specified time.

In the outpatient setting, it is the physician's responsibility to inform the patient when to take the medication. In most cases, it will coincide with the hospital administration directions of "in the morning."

Processing a Medication Order

Billing or patient profile errors usually occur in this step, and they can be dangerous or costly. The following step-by-step method helps to reduce the chance of error when entering and processing a prescription:

1. When pulling up a patient profile to begin entering a prescription, make sure the entire last name is spelled out and that the first letter of the first name is entered. When this is done, the computer will display a list of patients with that last name and the same first letter of the first name. Then you can choose which patient to fill it for by verifying the patient's date of birth.

2. Verify insurance information. This is done when the patient presents new insurance information.

3. Enter and select the physician the same way a patient is selected in step 1. If the wrong physician is put on the prescription, there is potential for an insurance audit or a pharmacist oversight resulting in an error.

4. Enter the medication to be dispensed. There are two ways this can be done: by NDC or by drug name. NDC (National Drug Code) is a standardized method used by all manufacturers to identify each individual drug by a sequence of numbers. All NDCs consist of 11 digits which appear in the format 12345-6789-10. The first five digits indicate the manufacturer, the next four digits indicate the drug and strength, and the last two digits indicate package size.

5. Enter the quantity to be dispensed, which may change due to a patient's insurance coverage. Most insurance companies cover only 30 days at a retail pharmacy.

6. Enter sig (direction) codes. This is where another vital mistake can occur. If the pharmacy technician interprets the prescription incorrectly, it will be typed and appear on the label incorrectly. If the pharmacist misses this mistake and dispenses it to a patient, then the patient will take the medication incorrectly and could possibly be harmed.

7. Enter the day supply. This is the total quantity divided by how many times a day the medication is to be used. For example: 90 tablets/TID = 30 days. Errors in this step can lead to an insurance audit.

8. Enter the exact number of refills on the prescription. The pharmacy technician must include this information, according to law.

9. Enter the expiration date, which comes directly from the stock bottle. If the wrong expiration date is entered, the patient could potentially take expired medication.

10. Process through insurance. This is the last step, where the pharmacy receives authorization to dispense a drug.

Patient Profiles

All pharmacies must maintain patient-specific profiles of medications dispensed to the patient. Originally, these were handwritten lists of medications dispensed, including dates, initials of the dispensing/recording pharmacists, the name and quantity of the drug, the prescribing physician, and any other pertinent data. Profiles include the patient's name, date of birth, address, drug allergies, and adverse reactions to drugs. The intent was for the pharmacist to review the patient's profile for allergies and possible drug interactions and to intercede for any contraindications, allergies, and/or duplication of therapy prior to the dispensing of the medication. However, in busy high-volume pharmacies, the documentation of the medication on the profile may occur after the patient has picked up the medication.

With the advent of the computer age and electronic pharmacy programs, patient profiles now contain insurance information, billing issues, information regarding particular prescriptions, and may even contain personal information as to who may pick up the medication or when a physician will authorize early refills. When processing a new prescription or refill, the pharmacy may directly interface with the insurance company, allowing instant access to payment, co-payment, and coverage issues. Many times the computer access may simply be the process of changing a non-formulary or expensive co-payment medication to one that is covered, or with a less expensive co-payment. The programs will screen for drug interactions, allergies, and therapeutic duplications and will flash warning screens during prescription entry, dispensing, and verification. This allows for multiple checks of any issues the computer has identified.

Residents of licensed healthcare facilities, such as nursing homes, usually have their medications dispensed by pharmacies utilizing outpatient computer programs. Patients in acute care facilities may have their medications dispensed by a stand-alone pharmacy system—a system that is connected to the hospital's billing and information system, or one that is contained within an integrated computer program. The degree of patient information the pharmacy must enter into the program is dependent upon the type of information flow between and among the systems. A stand-alone system requires total patient information input, while an integrated system may already have all of the information required. In an integrated system, the pharmacist may need to enter allergies, recent weights, or adverse drug events. Otherwise, the pharmacist has access to all of the information already collected for that patient, including transcribed physician admission reports, laboratory, radiology, and nursing reports, as well as home address, phone, insurance, and advanced directives. These systems are more complex but have the ability to screen more thoroughly for allergies, adverse reactions, contraindications, drug interactions, and food/drug interactions. They also have the ability to print notifications of drug therapy issues to the nursing floor, dietary team, and other designated recipients.

Computer patient profiles are also evolving into tools for all healthcare personnel. By integrating information with the patient's electronic record in his or her primary care physician's office, the hospital has access to reports and diagnoses prior to admission. The physician in the hospital can access his patient's office information. This facilitates patient care. Discussion has also begun between healthcare providers for the integration of the patient's retail pharmacy prescription information with physician's office information. Healthcare information is protected by federal law under the auspices of the Health Insurance Portability and Accountability Act. This legislation outlines the strict control and flow of health-related informa-tion between healthcare providers and was initiated to protect patients' healthcare privacy from undue examination by outside parties and any resulting discriminatory actions.

Purchasing and Inventory Control

Effective management of the drug inventory is necessary in all pharmacy practice settings. It is important that all staff understand the basic principles of managing the stock of drugs and participate actively in maintaining adequate inventory. Some staff may be more actively involved in inventory management. The involvement of technicians in inventory management is critical, and often a technician fills the specialized position of buyer, who is designated to do all inventory maintenance and ordering for a facility.

Inventory systems are organized to maintain an adequate supply of drugs at all times. They may be computerized systems that allow online drug purchases for just-in-time (JIT) arrival, track supply levels, and provide detailed reports on usage. Manual systems may be effective for smaller operations, but they require the same attention to specific detail that computerized systems automate. For example, manual systems might require posting of maximum and minimum levels as shelf labels rather than having them defined within the computer database.

The Formulary

A drug **formulary** is a continually revised list of drugs approved for purchase, stocking, and use at a facility or within a healthcare network. This list reflects the judgment of the hospital, pharmacy, medical staff, and the managed care or other third party payers. The purpose of the formulary is to improve the quality of care and control the costs associated with that care. At acute care facilities, a formulary is developed, maintained, and revised by the facility's pharmacy and therapeutics committee.

The formulary is used to determine product availability, including stocked dosage forms, strengths, and concentrations of medications. It may also contain advice on appropriate therapeutic uses of the approved drugs, state-acceptable dosage ranges, and policies regarding a drug's use or restrictions placed on the use of specific agents. Because the formulary defines the majority of drugs to be stocked, it serves as the reference for the pharmacy inventory.

However, there must be a method for obtaining non-formulary products required to meet patient needs. Usually a pharmacist determines when a non-formulary item is ordered. Non-formulary items commonly do not have an assigned storage location within the pharmacy, and unused portions may be returned. Non-formulary items may require a manual tracking system to monitor stock and determine the reorder point.

Inventory Control Systems

Inventory control must be organized in every pharmacy operation in order to maintain an adequate supply of drugs at all times. The control system facilitates ordering based on defined stocking levels. The point at which a drug is ordered is called the reorder point and is defined as the minimum stock level acceptable. The quantity to be ordered is defined by the difference between the quantities of product on hand and the **periodic automatic replenishment (PAR)** level, which is defined as the maximum level of product stocked. This process may be accomplished manually or by a computer.

A computerized inventory management system requires all transactions to be recorded in a computer. This is made easier if ordering is done online. Order points may be automated within this type of system, or may be initiated as needed. The computerized inventory management system has extensive reporting capability, including use by therapeutic category, product turnover rates, and maintenance of a perpetual inventory.

A manual inventory management system requires all transactions to be executed by hand. Reorder points and PAR levels are usually posted at the product storage location. Staff keeps track of what must be ordered by writing the information in an order book or on a "want list." It becomes critical for every item to be listed using this method, or stock will not be replaced in a timely manner. Writing down complete descriptive information, including strength, size, and dosage form, is critical for the buyer to be able to order the correct items.

A just-in-time inventory system is managed so that drugs arrive just before they are needed. This method minimizes investment in available stock by purchasing only when a drug is needed, maintaining inventory at minimal levels. However, this method does not work for all drugs because pharmacies must stock some items that are used infrequently or not at all. It also does not work well if staff fails to communicate high usage to the buyer.

Ordering Medications

The order can be communicated via a variety of methods, including telephone, fax, Internet, U.S. post, or directly to the sales representative or the vendor. Every order is initiated by completing a **purchase order** (PO), which is a business form that records the details of the order. Every PO includes the following information:

- purchase order number (PO #)
- name of the company
- date of the order
- product ordered
- quantity ordered
- price
- payment terms
- shipping address

An invoice is the bill of sale for products delivered and must be verified against the PO for accuracy. In addition, this document requests payment to the vendor.

Direct Purchasing

Direct purchasing is the execution of a PO between the pharmacy and the drug manufacturer without going through a drug wholesaler. Usually, this type of purchase involves items such as vaccines, drugs with special storage or shipping requirements, drugs in limited supply, or orphan drugs, which are drugs used for rare disease states.

Purchasing from Drug Wholesalers

Most pharmacies purchase the majority of their stock from a drug wholesaler. This method is also known as *prime vendor purchasing* because the wholesaler acts as the principle source of inventory. Purchasing from a prime vendor allows the pharmacy to acquire drugs from different manufacturers through a single vendor (the drug wholesaler), receive the order in a single delivery, and pay a single invoice. In order to have a contract with a prime vendor, the pharmacy must usually agree to buy 80 to 85% of its drugs from that single wholesale company.

Receiving Medications

Two of the most important parts of the pharmacy operation are the receipt and storage of stock into inventory. A poorly organized and executed system can put patients at risk and raise costs. Receiving and storing stock are a very useful training experiences for new employees because it teaches them the formulary, helps them learn product appearance, and shows them the correct storage locations within the department.

The receiving process verifies that the shipment is complete and intact before putting it into storage and use. The person receiving the shipment completes the receiving process and must document any abnormalities and discrepancies on the shipping manifest or refuse shipment. The receiving process includes verification of the "ship to" name and address on containers; verification that the number of boxes matches the courier's shipping manifest; inspection of each box for gross damage; checking products received against the receiving copy of the

PO; and signing, dating, and filing a copy of the PO or receiving slip.

In order to determine that the product matches the PO, the person receiving the delivery must verify that all of the following are correct:

- name of item
- brand of item
- dosage form
- size of package
- concentration or strength
- quantity of product

In addition, the person receiving the shipment must check each product's expiration date for adequate shelf life. Any staff member who removes an item before it is checked into inventory must leave a note indicating the removal so that the delivery can be reconciled.

The storing process places drugs received into proper storage locations. Products requiring refrigeration or freezing should be processed first. It is very important to maintain proper stock rotation. When placing inventory into storage, compare expiration dates and place earliest to expire in front, remove any stock that has expired, and highlight products having a short shelf life with a small tag showing the upcoming expiration date.

Technicians spend more time handling and preparing drugs than pharmacists, and therefore have a critical responsibility to assess and evaluate products for content and labeling to confirm that the receiving and storing processes have been done properly.

Products Requiring Special Handling

Controlled Substances

There are specific ordering, receiving, storage, dispensing, inventory, record keeping, returning, wasting, and disposal requirements for controlled substances. Transactions for this class of item are DEA-regulated with respect to ordering or record keeping, and registration with the DEA is required to purchase or distribute these items. **DEA Form 222** is required documentation for every transaction that includes schedule II controlled substances.

DEA Form 222 is used to order schedule CII drugs. Execution of this form is restricted to the primary staff member registered with the DEA; only this registrant, or someone given power of attorney by this registrant, may sign the order form. The forms are issued in triplicate copies, with copy one retained by the supplier, copy two sent to the DEA, and copy three retained and filed by the pharmacy. A supplier may partially fill an order on a DEA Form 222 provided the remainder is filled within 60 days.

The person completing DEA Form 222 must complete it using a typewriter, pen, or indelible pencil. Each order form has ten lines, and only one item can be ordered per line. The signature must match that of the registrant or person with power of attorney. There can be no erasures or strikeouts on the form. The number of containers received and the date of receipt must be written on copy three of DEA Form 222 and the forms kept on file (filed separately from other pharmacy records and readily retrievable) for a minimum of two years. Many pharmacies file DEA Form 222 stapled to the corresponding invoice in this filed location. These forms must be ordered directly from the DEA. Special order forms are not required for ordering schedule CIII through CV substances.

Records must be kept of the initial and subsequent inventories of controlled drugs and their receipt, dispensing, and disposal. Upon discovery, a loss or theft must be reported on DEA Form 106.

Expired controlled drugs may not be returned to manufacturer, but must be destroyed, with the destruction documented on a special DEA form. A DEA-sanctioned company should complete the actual disposal, and the form should be completed and submitted to the DEA immediately after disposal occurs. A DEA representative will sign and return a copy of the form to the pharmacy for their records.

Investigational Drugs

Investigational drugs are medications that are used in human clinical trials before a drug is marketed. These drugs are being tested for safety and effectiveness. Investigational drugs require special ordering, inventorying, and handling procedures. The primary investigating physician usually orders the products, but the pharmacy often manages the inventory using perpetual inventory records. Expired investigational drugs must not be destroyed, but instead have to be returned to the study sponsor with every dose accounted for.

Compounded Products

Products compounded by the pharmacy, including oral liquids, topicals, or sterile products, must have expiration dates monitored closely. These products usually have much shorter expirations ranging from days to months rather than years. These products cannot be returned because there is no manufacturer in the conventional sense. They must be disposed of in accordance with pharmacy policy, state, and federal regulations.

Repackaged Pharmaceuticals

Unit dose tablets, capsules, and oral liquids are some bulk packages that may be **repackaged** by the pharmacy. The expiration dates of these products must be monitored closely because they have expiration dating that has been reassigned due to the repackaging process. The new expiration dating is one year (with proper packaging materials) or the manufacturer's listed expiration date, whichever comes first. Products that have been repackaged cannot be returned to the original manufacturer and must be disposed of in accordance with policy and regulations.

Medication Distribution Systems

Acute Setting

There are two distribution systems that are typically used in the acute, or institutional, setting. The appropriate system will be chosen based on a variety of factors—size of facility, number of patients, and severity of patient medication needs.

Centralized Pharmacy

When pharmacy services are **centralized**, all services are provided from a single physical location within a facility. This means that all functional areas are within the same room or contiguous rooms. Often, this is the choice when services or resources are limited, as with a small facility. In a centralized pharmacy, the unit dose fill station, the outpatient pharmacy, and all storage for drugs and supplies are located together. A centralized pharmacy may also have a **clean room** where intravenous solutions are made in a sterile environment. The clean room includes **high efficiency particulate air (HEPA) filters** that will remove any particle, including bacteria, greater than 0.22 microns.

Centralized organization is often chosen because this is the most cost-effective manner of staffing; it requires fewer people for all services when they are all in one room. There are several disadvantages to centralizing services, however. There is often a lack of face-to-face interaction with patients and other hospital staff, and it takes more time to deliver drugs to the areas where they are needed.

In a centralized pharmacy, technicians are responsible for preparing the IV and other sterile solutions, filling the medication carts, filling floor stock or medications, filling IV solutions that are stored on nursing units for convenience purposes, filling and delivering narcotic orders, compounding and repackaging extemporaneously, billing for services provided, and managing quality control and improvement.

Decentralized Pharmacy

Decentralized pharmacy services are used in conjunction with a central pharmacy but are provided from within a patient care area of the hospital, such as a nursing unit or intensive care unit. The most common form is a satellite pharmacy—an area designated to serve specific patient care services, such as an oncology unit. Drugs for patients in this specific area are stored, prepared, and dispensed from the satellite which is staffed by a pharmacist and often a pharmacy technician.

The advantages of a decentralized pharmacy service are proximity to patient care areas, access to pharmacy information by other staff, ease of monitoring patient responses to therapy, and sharing of educational materials. The disadvantages are that it requires additional staff, resources, and drug inventory.

The responsibilities of a technician in a pharmacy satellite vary by institution. If they are present in a satellite, technicians help the pharmacists to provide care, help maintain drug inventory, prepare both oral and IV doses, and answer staff questions.

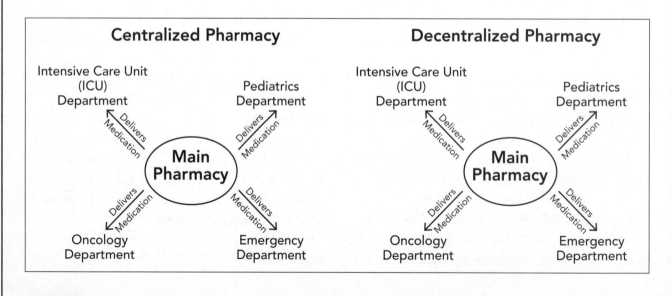

Unit Dose System

The **unit dose** (UD) system of medication distribution is a pharmacy-coordinated method of dispensing and controlling medications in organized healthcare settings. This system has become almost universal as a technique of providing medications to patients in acute care facilities. In this system, each dose of a medication is packaged in a single (unit) package. Each package is labeled with all required information and remains sealed until administration.

Using this system, the pharmacy has to dispense a more limited supply of medications each day. These drugs are usually contained in a medication cart or automated dispensing cabinet on the nursing unit. If not used, each package may be returned to the pharmacy and dispensed later to the same or a different patient.

Home-Care Setting

A home-care setting is where the administration of medication is given in the home. There are many reasons why a patient would opt for this choice, including end-of-life care, increased privacy, or even a sense of security during treatment. The technician plays a vital role in the preparation of medications for these patients.

Home-Care IV Admixures

One of the most important specialized services provided by a home-care pharmacy is an intravenous (IV) admixture program. Home-care pharmacies must follow the same compounding laws and standards as pharmacies in a hospital. Each facility must ensure that it establishes **quality assurance** (QA) and **quality control** (QC) policies and procedures to maintain the highest quality of compounded product. The mandated standards for sterile compounding address each of these activities and are stipulated by the United States Pharmacopoeia (USP) chapter 797 or USP 797.

Home-Care Infusion Systems

A home-care pharmacy uses many of the same intravenous therapeutic modalities as those in an acute care environment. There are various types of IV delivery methods related to the acute care setting, including gravity feed, rate-restricted IV administration sets, and **infusion** pumps for large or mini-bags or syringe infusion pumps for syringe doses.

Medication Errors

Pharmacists and technicians are responsible for the safe and appropriate use of medications in all pharmacy practice settings. As part of the healthcare team, the role of the pharmacist is to cooperatively establish patient-specific drug therapy regimens designed to achieve predefined therapeutic outcomes without subjecting the patient to undue risk of harm.

When an error reaches a patient, it is frequently because multiple breakdowns have occurred in the drug ordering, distribution, and administration systems. Often, more than one thing has gone wrong. Someone's lack of knowledge or substandard performance has slipped through the drug distribution system safety net undetected. This occurs when caregivers circumvent the system or when they do not give safety checks and balances a chance to function. In some situations, an adequate system is not present.

There are many types of errors in dispensing medications.

Prescribing Errors

Prescribing errors occur when the drug is ordered incorrectly, patient characteristics are not considered, or the order is illegible.

Omissions

Omission errors occur when an ordered dose is not administered. Omission errors do not include if the patient cannot take the drug, it is prior to a procedure, the caregiver is waiting for lab results, or the patient refuses to take the medication.

Wrong Time

Wrong time errors occur when the drug is administered too early or too late. Hospitals often have predetermined administration time set by policy, and an acceptable interval may be within a 30-minute window of the official administration time. Drugs given outside this window are considered an error.

Unauthorized Drug

If a drug is given without a prescriber order, given to the wrong patient, shared among family members at home, refilled without authorization, or administered outside an approved protocol, it is an unauthorized drug.

Improper Dose

Improper dose errors occur when a patient is given more or less than the prescribed amount. Doses that cannot be accurately measured are excluded, as are the variances in converting between systems of measure.

Wrong Dosage Form

If doses are administered or dispensed in a form that differs from what is ordered, a wrong dosage form error occurs. However, depending upon state law or facility guidelines, it may be acceptable to modify the dosage form to accommodate patient needs.

Wrong Drug Preparation

Drug preparation errors occur when a drug is reconstituted with an incorrect volume of water, if bacteriostatic saline is used in place of sterile water for injection, if the seal is not broken on a ready-to-mix product, or if the wrong base product is used when compounding an ointment or cream.

Wrong Administration Technique

Administration errors occur when doses are given using an inappropriate procedure or technique. For example, subcutaneous injection given too deep, IV infused by gravity instead of by infusion pump, or eye or ear drops are instilled into the incorrect location.

Deteriorated Drug

Drugs given after their expiration date may have lost their potency, or they may have deteriorated into toxic compounds. The same may be true of drugs given after improper storage. Dispensing such drugs is a deteriorated drug error.

Monitoring

Monitoring errors occur when drug therapy is not reviewed adequately. This may occur if drug levels were not ordered when required, ordered levels were not reviewed, the caregiver did not respond to levels reported to be outside the therapeutic range, the blood pressure was not measured when an antihypertensive drug was given, or blood sugar was not measured when a hypoglycemic drug was ordered.

Compliance

When patients fail to adhere to a prescribed drug regimen, compliance errors occur. This is evident when refill requests come too early or too late, when the patient fails to understand instructions for use of their medications, when side effects become intolerable, or if the cost of the prescription is more than the patient can afford.

Continuous Quality Improvement

Continuous quality improvement is a management system that attempts to understand the service process, identify problem areas, and establish specific, measurable expectations to improve quality in the future.

Quality Assurance (QA)

Quality assurance is a program of activities that ensure the procedures used in the preparation of compounded products lead to a product that meets certain standards.

A QA program should include:

- A documented, ongoing QA program for training, monitoring, and evaluating pharmacy personnel performance. This ensures that each member understands what is required of them and is adhering to the standard set forth.

- A documented, ongoing QA program for testing and monitoring equipment used in compounding. This is required to ensure that all equipment used in the preparation of these products is working properly and at its highest efficiency.
- A documented, ongoing QA program for monitoring and testing the compounded products. This helps to identify if all other QA programs are working properly.
- A documented, ongoing QA program for monitoring and evaluating patient outcomes to ensure efficacy of the compounded products. This ensures that the products dispensed from the pharmacy are treating the patient properly.
- A written plan for corrective measures if problems are identified by the QA audits. This ensures that deficiencies in the QA plan are identified and corrected.
- QA activities are put through a documented, periodic review for effectiveness.

Quality Control

Quality control is a set of testing activities used to determine the quality of compounded products, which works in conjunction with the quality assurance plan. The tests focus on ingredients, devices or components, and the final prepared product to determine whether they meet required standards. In general, quality control is the daily management of quality within the pharmacy. It should include the following:

- a standard operating procedure to document the calibration and maintenance of equipment being used to compound prescriptions
- a standard operating procedure to document pharmacy personnel training and validation
- a standard operating procedure for product recalls

- a standard operating procedure to document monitoring of the compounding environments, both sterile and non-sterile
- a standard operating procedure to evaluate, confirm, and document the quality of the final compounded product

The Hospital Setting

As mentioned earlier, the roles of pharmacy technicians vary depending on the pharmacy setting. Thus far, we have focused primarily on the retail setting, but the national exam will also have questions concerning the hospital setting—which is as different as night and day to the retail setting.

This section of this chapter will go over different roles required of the pharmacy technician in the hospital setting. This includes individual patient cassette filling, providing a 24-hour supply of unit dose (individual packaged) medication for individual patients, and the making of individual IV admixtures. A basic understanding of principles involved in the filling of medication orders/IV admixtures is critical in ensuring not only the correct medication but also, in the case of IV admixtures, in ensuring no contamination has occurred that could harm the patient. With this in mind, this section will also go over the importance of aseptic technique.

Working in the Hospital Setting

The hospital setting involves the treatment of patients who have been admitted. Oral medications and IV admixtures are integral parts of treating these patients until they are healthy enough to be discharged from the hospital setting. In some cases, patients will be around for only a short time, receiving treatment for a type of acute (short term) condition or disease state, or for a very long time, receiving treatment for a chronic (long term) condition or disease state. Your role as the pharmacy technician is to ensure that medication and IV admixture orders are prepared correctly, as you will be the one filling 95% of these orders.

The hospital setting generally has two sections that allow them to fill medication orders and IV admixtures. Medication orders are filled in what is known as the cassette filling area, where medications are filled in individual cassettes with a 24-hour supply. A **cassette** is a small boxed unit/drawer with spaces in which to place medication, and it will have the patient's name written in the front. Each cassette is reserved for one individual patient and fits into a cart of many cassettes for multiple patients on a unit or ward. Unlike in the retail setting, medications used are what we call unit dose medication, which can be purchased from the drug manufacturer or prepared in the pharmacy setting as a pre-pack.

Unit Dose Medications

A unit dose is a drug that is individually prepackaged. A unit dose will have the drug name, strength, manufacturer, expiration date, and lot number. It is important when filling the individual cassette tray that the unit dose medication match what is ordered to a computer printout list of medications the patient is on. Unit dose medication can be individual oral tablets, capsules, or oral liquid formulations such as a suspension and, in some cases, injections.

Each inpatient pharmacy has its own timetable for what is called a cart exchange. A cart exchange is when a cart holding patient medication cassettes is replaced with a new 24-hour supply of patient medication cassettes. Cart exchange occurs once a day, or every 24 hours at the same time each day.

Working in the cassette area is an intricate part of providing patient care, as it is important that the right 24-hour supply of medications is placed in each individual cassette correctly. Most hospitals will have the pharmacist check the technician's work, but some have begun what is known as a tech-check-tech program, where another technician checks the filled cassettes. A study showed this method to be more effective in reducing medication errors than having a pharmacist checking the technicians' work.

The Pyxis® Machine

The **Pyxis®** machine is similar to a candy vending machine, where issuing drugs is automated simply by pushing a button. Some hospital settings have done away with cassette filling and are now being fully automated with Pyxis® machines, while some use both methods in the distribution of patient medications.

The Pyxis® machine can be fully automated in the hospital pharmacy setting to allow the distribution of hundreds of medications, or it can be simplified to distribute 50 or fewer medications. For the lower-yield Pyxis® machines, you would find these in nursing units for nurses to use in dispensing medication to individual patients.

The role of the pharmacy technician is to ensure that the drawers/bins that contain medications in these machines are filled correctly. This in itself can be a full-time job, as many checks are needed to ensure the drawer has the correct medication in it. Pyxis® machines, also known as Omnicell® machines depending on the company that make them, also allow for the billing of patients who receive medications and, in some cases, will inform a nurse when a medication is due for a patient.

The other aspect of the hospital pharmacy setting is the **IV room**, where IV solutions and other sterile products are prepared.

The IV Room

The IV room is usually a separate room that contains IV supplies, as well as **laminar flow hoods** that provide a clean environment in the making of IV or sterile products. There are two types of laminar flow hoods: the horizontal, or general, hood is used to prepare sterile products like IV solutions. The vertical, or chemo, hood is used in the preparation of hazardous drugs, such as chemo drugs for cancer patients or drugs derived from human blood. Today, both hoods are kept on 24-hours a day, seven days a week, but if for some reason the hood has been turned off, you must wait at least 30 minutes before using it.

Each laminar flow hood has two filters. The first filter is what we call a particulate filter, which will take out any particles in the air that are greater than five microns (such as dust). The second filter is called the high efficiency particulate air (HEPA) filter, which will take out any particles greater than 0.22 to 0.3 microns (which is the size of the smallest bacteria). Laminar flow hood service should be performed every six months to ensure all is working well, and also to replace HEPA filters if needed.

The cleaning of both laminar flow hoods should be done with **isopropyl alcohol 70%** or greater. Cleaning of the hood should be done before use, during use as needed, and after use. Proper cleaning involves wiping with a clean cloth and using isopropyl alcohol 70% from back to front of hood, using side-to-side motions away from the HEPA filter.

In preparing your **IV admixture** or sterile product, it is imperative that you only have inside the hood what you need to prepare. All items should be in a horizontal line to ensure the HEPA filter air flow goes around your items. You should work at least six inches inside the hood.

Some hospitals' clean rooms are actually one big laminar flow hood, with several HEPA filters throughout the room. In this case, you actually need to wear personal protective equipment (PPE) such as mask, gloves, and gown before entering the clean room. There are many protocols established for working in the clean room to ensure you have not contaminated the product you are making. Recently, the making of sterile products has become a big issue with the FDA, and guidelines in the *United States Pharmacopeia* (which deals with standards) has a whole chapter (USP 797) dealing with this topic.

As mentioned, in the preparation of IV admixtures or sterile products it is important to ensure correct medication, etc., but it is also important to ensure that you have not contaminated the IV, potentially causing harm to the patient. Realize that an IV goes directly into the patient's body.

Aseptic Technique

The importance of aseptic technique cannot be overstated, as you do not want to introduce a pathogen (disease-causing microorganism) into the IV being prepared. Aseptic technique is preparing a sterile product without contaminating it. The first step of aseptic technique, or infection control, is to wash your hands correctly and frequently! The use of aseptic technique also involves the practical (hands-on) experience of preparing IVs or sterile products without contaminating them. Learning techniques and knowing what to touch/not touch are critical to ensure a safe product is running through the veins of a patient.

IV Room Supplies

Some of the tools used in the IV room include the syringe, needle, IV bags, additive **vials**, **ampules**, and lots of isopropyl alcohol 70% swipe pads.

- Syringe: a unit that holds IV drugs you will inject into an IV bag. It consists of three parts, which include the barrel (which indicates measurements), the plunger (which is how you remove medication from an admixture vial or push the medication into the IV bag), and the tip (which will have a special **luer lock** to hold the needle in place). Syringes come in different sizes based on volume, from the 1 ml tuberculin syringe to the 60 ml syringe.
- Needle: allows you to pierce the admixture vial for removal of drug into the syringe or allows you to pierce the IV bag to deliver medication to the IV bag. Needles come in different sizes based on the **gauge** (G) of the needle; the lower the gauge, the bigger the bore (diameter) of the needle. The length of the needle depends on how long you want your needle to be to make it easier to withdraw or add necessary contents of the syringe.
- IV bags: mostly made of plastic due to easy storage and cost. Some IV solutions still come in glass bottles, as certain medications will leach into a plastic bag. Sizes range from 50 ml to 1,000 ml

in volume, but in some cases you will see larger-volume IV bags. An IV bag has two ports: one for introduction of medication with a needle/syringe and one that connects to the IV line which goes into the patient. Always remember to clean the port using isopropyl alcohol 70% pads before introducing medication into that port.

- Additive vials: come in sizes ranging from 2 ml to usually 50 ml. A vial will either be single-dose, which is meant for the withdrawal of just one dose before the vial is discarded, or multi-dose, which is meant to be pierced by a needle for multiple doses. A vial will have the medication name on it, as well as necessary information like concentration, stability, usage directions, expiration date, and lot number, etc.

Some vials will come in a powder formulation and will need to have diluents (solution) added before administration. The rationale for powder vials is that the stability of the drug is short; and once diluents are added, it will have a very short expiration date. The addition of a diluent to a powder vial is called **reconstitution**. The vial will give information as to which diluents should be added and how much is needed to attain a specific concentration. Always remember to clean the port using isopropyl alcohol 70% pads before piercing the rubber (diaphragm) top of the vial.

- Ampules: self-enclosed glass containers that contain sterile drugs for injection into an IV bag. Ampules can easily be opened at the neck (top) of the ampule, but removal of their contents must be done by a **filter needle or straw**. Once medication is removed, then the filter needle or straw must be replaced with a regular needle before injecting it into an IV bag. The rationale for using the filter needle or straw is that once an ampule is broken, it will leave microscopic glass shards. The filter needle or straw will take out anything greater than five microns.

IV bags come in different sizes and are used for either fluid and/or electrolyte replacement in the administration of medication or drugs. **Large volume parenterals** (LVP) are around 500 ml to 1,000 ml, while **small volume parenterals** (SVP) are around 250 ml to 500 ml. Both of these are used for the delivery of fluid or **electrolytes**. Generally, an LVP would be used for an adult, while an SVP would be used for a pediatric patient. The infusion rate of both types of IVs is dependent on the patient, but generally is set for hours. Infusion is the injection of a large volume of fluid over a prolonged period of time. Electrolytes are the most common IV ingredients, including potassium (K), sodium (Na), chloride (Cl), and magnesium (Mg), as these all carry an electric charge and are important for the body.

IV SOLUTION	ABBREVIATION	WHAT IS IN IT
dextrose 5% water	D5W	5 g dextrose in 100 ml sterile water
0.9% NaCl	normal saline (NS)	0.9 g NaCl in 100 ml sterile water
0.45% NaCl	$\frac{1}{2}$ NS	0.45 g NaCl in 100 ml sterile water
0.22% NaCl	$\frac{1}{4}$ NS	0.225 g NaCl in 100 ml sterile water
D5%/0.9% NaCl	D5NS	5 g dextrose and 0.9% NaCl in 100 ml sterile water
D5%/0.45% NaCl	D5 $\frac{1}{2}$ NS	5 g dextrose and 0.45% NaCl in 100 ml sterile water

Small-volume IV bags hold around 50 to 250 ml, with 50 ml as the most common size for administering medication or drugs. They are called **intravenous piggy backs** (IVPB) because the small-volume bag delivers the medication into a running IV line, or piggy backs the IV line. The **flow rate** (how long an IV is to run until completion) of an IVPB is usually between 30 and 60 minutes.

Total Parenteral Nutrition

Another type of IV is total parenteral nutrition (TPN), which is used for those who are unable to take anything by mouth after an operation or because they are resting the digestive system. A TPN, also known as a hyperalimentation, is made up of many ingredients, such as dextrose (which is broken down into glucose in the body), **aminosyn** (for amino acids or protein), **lipids** (fats), electrolytes, vitamins, minerals, etc. The use of a TPN is essentially to replace feeding that would normally be done by mouth. Because there are many potential ingredients involved in the preparation of a TPN, it is imperative that the pharmacy technician understand his/her role in its preparation, including the importance of aseptic technique.

The importance of working in the IV room cannot be overstated, as technicians fill 95% of all IV admixture orders. Many may already be prepared by the manufacturer, requiring only that a label be attached, but there will also be situations where one or more **additives** will be needed, as well as powdered drugs that need to be reconstituted first.

The development of good aseptic technique is vital to ensure that an IV is made without contamination. This involves learning the skills necessary and developing habits that allow aseptic technique to be followed at all times when preparing not only IV admixtures, but any sterile product.

Practice Questions

1. Which of the following standards does the preparation of IV admixtures need to adhere to?
   a. USP 795
   b. USP 797
   c. OSHA
   d. FDA

2. Which would be considered a false statement when referring to the policy and procedures manual?
   a. Policies and procedures also promote safety in the workplace.
   b. They are a compilation of previous decisions made that define the way the pharmacy will operate.
   c. Policies and procedures also serve as the basis for the training of new staff.
   d. There is no false statement, as all of the above are correct.

3. Which of the following items would not be found in the *policy and procedures* manual?
   a. operations standards
   b. accreditation standards
   c. BOP regulations concerning pharmacy technicians
   d. how to fill a prescription

4. In which of the following settings are medication orders utilized?
   a. hospital inpatient
   b. hospital outpatient
   c. retail
   d. none of the above

5. What is the minimum, mandated amount of time for maintaining medication order records?
   a. one year
   b. three years
   c. five years
   d. ten years

6. Which of the following methods is NOT a way that an outpatient prescription can be presented to a pharmacy?
   a. handwritten by the prescriber on a preprinted prescription form
   b. computer-generated and sent to the pharmacy via fax
   c. pneumatic tube
   d. electronically communicated to the pharmacy from computer to computer

7. Which of the following methods is NOT a part of interpreting a medication order?
   a. reviewing the order for clarity
   b. identifying the patient
   c. selecting the drug product
   d. scheduling medication times

8. When processing a prescription, which information should be used to verify that the drug product is correct?
   a. medication name
   b. medication strength
   c. NDC number
   d. manufacturer

9. Which of the following pieces of information would NOT be considered part of the patient's profile?
   a. date of birth
   b. address
   c. name
   d. primary physician

10. What is the name of the list of approved medications for purchasing, stocking, and use in a given facility?
    a. inventory
    b. stock
    c. formulary
    d. PAR

11. What does PAR stand for?
    a. periodic automatic review
    b. peer-assisted review
    c. partially automated replenishment
    d. periodic automated replenishment

12. Which of the following items is listed on a purchase order?
    a. date of order
    b. product ordered
    c. payment terms
    d. all of the above

13. Which of the following terms is defined as a pharmacy purchasing from the drug manufacturer?
    a. direct purchasing
    b. group purchasing
    c. wholesale purchasing
    d. none of the above

14. Which of the following items is NOT verified when checking in an order for medication?
    a. name of item
    b. storage directions
    c. package size
    d. quantity

15. Which of the following medications is DEA Form 222 used to order?
    a. CIV controlled substances
    b. CII controlled substances
    c. CV controlled substances
    d. CIII controlled substances

16. Which of the following locations is classified as a pharmacy that provides services from a single location?
    a. decentralized pharmacy
    b. chain pharmacy
    c. centralized pharmacy
    d. none of the above

17. If a medication is packaged as a unit dose, how many items will be packaged together?
    a. one
    b. three
    c. five
    d. six or more

18. If a medication order is illegible and the wrong medication is dispensed as a result, what type of error is that considered?
    a. wrong time
    b. improper dose
    c. unauthorized drug
    d. prescribing error

19. Which of the following types of prescriptions are not refillable?
    a. CIV controlled substances
    b. CIII controlled substances
    c. CII controlled substances
    d. CV controlled substances

20. Which of the following terms is defined as a program of activities used to ensure procedures meet a set standard?
    a. policy
    b. procedure
    c. quality assurance
    d. quality control

21. Which of the following terms is defined as testing activities used to determine the quality of a product?
    a. policy
    b. procedure
    c. quality assurance
    d. quality control

22. What is the typical turnaround time for a medication to be filled in the hospital setting?
   a. 1–2 hours
   b. 2–4 hours
   c. 6–12 hours
   d. 24 hours

23. Which of the following notations indicates the urgency of a medication order?
   a. STAT
   b. ASAP
   c. NOW
   d. all of the above

24. Which of the following items on a medication order should be checked to ensure completeness?
   a. date
   b. patient name
   c. medication name
   d. all of the above

25. Any question regarding a protocol for a specific action, such as a recall of a drug or how to return expired drugs, would be found in what manual?
   a. pharmacy practice book
   b. pharmacy procedures manual
   c. *United States Pharmacopea Volume I*
   d. *Facts and Comparisons*

26. The use of a filter needle or filter straw is necessary when using what following unit?
   a. single-dose vial
   b. multi-dose vial
   c. ampule
   d. syringe with a luer lock tip

27. Of the following IVs, which one would be used for the administration of medication?
   a. SVP
   b. LVP
   c. IVPB
   d. TPN

28. LVPs and SVPs are generally used for
   a. fluid replacement.
   b. electrolyte replacement.
   c. both fluid and electrolyte replacement.
   d. medication.

29. As the gauge of a needle increases,
   a. the length of the needle increases as well.
   b. the diameter of the needle increases as well.
   c. the length of the needle decreases.
   d. the diameter of the needle decreases.

30. The term *reconstitution* applies to which of the following?
   a. the single-dose vial
   b. the multi-dose vial
   c. the ampule
   d. a powdered vial

31. A filter needle will remove contents greater than
   a. 0.22 microns.
   b. two microns.
   c. five microns.
   d. ten microns.

32. What is the proper technique in the cleaning of a laminar flow hood?
   a. Wipe from back to front using side-to-side motions, away from the HEPA filter.
   b. Wipe toward the HEPA filter and back continuously until the whole hood is cleaned.
   c. Wipe up and down along the sides of the hood and the back of the hood.
   d. There is no need to clean the hood, as it is self-cleaning.

33. You have D5W 500 ml running over four hours; for how many milliliters per minute should you set your administration pump?
   a. approximately 1 ml per minute
   b. approximately 2 ml per minute
   c. approximately 3 ml per minute
   d. approximately 4 ml per minute

34. What is the normal rate of administration for an IVPB?
   a. 10 to 20 minutes
   b. 30 to 60 minutes
   c. 60 to 90 minutes
   d. 90 to 180 minutes

35. Cassettes should contain how many hours' supply of medication?
   a. 12 hours
   b. 24 hours
   c. 36 hours
   d. 48 hours

36. What recent special guidelines should be following in the preparation of sterile products?
   a. DEA Form 222
   b. USP 254
   c. USP 797
   d. *Handbook of Injectable Drugs*

37. Which of the following statements is false?
   a. A unit dose is a drug that is individually prepackaged.
   b. Aseptic technique is preparing a sterile product without contaminating it.
   c. The vertical hood is used in the preparation of all sterile IV solutions.
   d. The laminar flow hood's HEPA filter will take out any particles greater than 0.3 microns.

38. Sometimes it is necessary to use personal protective equipment. Which of the following is considered to be PPE?
   a. glass plate to ensure you do not come into contact with what you are making
   b. clothing, such as masks, gowns, shoe covers, and gloves
   c. another technician to help you prepare sterile products
   d. a portable HEPA filter

39. Which needle has the largest diameter?
   a. 3 ml 25 G$\frac{1}{2}$"
   b. 5 ml 25 G1"
   c. 10 ml 25 G1$\frac{1}{2}$"
   d. They all have the same diameter.

40. If the laminar flow hood is turned off, how long should you wait to use it once turned on?
   a. 0 minutes
   b. 10 minutes
   c. 20 minutes
   d. 30 minutes

Answers and Explanations

1. b. USP 797 establishes standards for the preparation of IV admixtures. USP 795 addresses non-sterile compounding, OSHA oversees workplace safety, and the FDA oversees drugs on the market.

2. d. All statements made are correct. Policies and procedures promote safety in the workplace, are a compilation of previous decisions made that define the way the pharmacy will operate, and also serve as the basis for training new staff.

3. c. Board of pharmacy list of regulations for pharmacy technicians would not be a part of the pharmacy policy and procedures manual.

4. a. Medication orders are only utilized in the hospital setting.

5. b. The pharmacy must maintain medication order records for a minimum of three years.

6. c. The pneumatic tube system is only used in the institutional setting.

7. a. Reviewing the order for clarity is part of receiving the order, not part of interpreting a medication order process. Identifying the patient, selecting the drug product, and scheduling medication times are all part of the medication order process.

8. c. The NDC number should always be used to identify the drug product to be dispensed. Although the product can be verified using the medication name, the medication strength, and the manufacturer, the NDC is the most effective way to ensure that all information about the drug product is correct.

9. d. The patient profile will contain only patient demographic information.

10. c. The formulary is the list of approved medications. Inventory and stock are both items found in the pharmacy, and PAR identifies the level of inventory that will initiate an automatic reorder of a medication.

11. d. PAR stands for periodic automated replenishment.

12. d. All of the items—date of order, product ordered, and payment terms—will be found on the purchase order.

13. a. Direct purchasing is when a pharmacy purchases directly from a manufacturer. Group purchasing is when a collection of pharmacies purchase together. Wholesale purchasing is when a pharmacy purchases from a wholesaler.

14. b. The storage directions do not need to be checked to verify a product has been received, but the name of the item, the package size, and the quantity do need to be checked.

15. b. DEA Form 222 is used to order CII controlled substances. All other controlled substances can be ordered without using this form.

16. c. A centralized pharmacy offers services from a single location. Decentralized and chain pharmacies offer services in multiple locations.

17. a. A unit dose is packaged as a single unit.

18. d. A prescribing error results from an illegible prescription. A wrong time error occurs when a medication is given at an improper time. An improper dose error occurs when the medication given is correct but at a wrong dose. Unauthorized drug errors occur when the medication is given without a physician's order.

19. c. CII controlled substances cannot be refilled, while CIV, CIII, and CV can be refilled up to a maximum of five times if the physician indicates that.

20. c. Quality assurance is the activities used to verify that procedures meet a set standard.

21. d. Quality control is the process of testing activities that validate the QA process.

22. a. Typically, a medication should be filled and dispensed to the patient within one to two hours of receiving the order.

23. d. All of these notations—STAT, ASAP, and NOW—indicate an urgency.

24. d. All of the items—date, patient name, and medication name—are necessary for a medication order to be considered complete.

25. b. The pharmacy procedures manual would be where one would look first to see if there is an established protocol as to what should be done in a given situation.

26. c. The ampule is a self-enclosed, single-dose glass container that can be easily broken for removal of contents, but does require a filter needle or straw to ensure that all glass shards are removed as well.

27. c. Intravenous piggybacks are used for the administration of medications. SVPs and LVPs are used for fluid and/or electrolyte replacement, and TPN is used to provide full nutritional value, as it contains all that is necessary for a patient who cannot take anything by mouth.

28. c. Both are used for fluid and/or electrolyte replacement. A large volume parenteral is generally used for adult patients, while a small volume parenteral would be most likely used for a pediatric patient.

29. d. As the gauge of a needle increases, the diameter (or bore) of the needle decreases.

30. d. Reconsititution involves the adding of a diluent (solution) to make a powder vial into a liquid formulation with a specific concentration. Always look on the vial or package insert for directions as to which diluent to use and the amount needed as well.

31. c. A filter needle or straw should take out anything that is greater than five microns. The HEPA filter in a laminar flow hood would take out anything greater than 0.22 microns.

32. a. The proper technique in the cleaning of a laminar flow hood would be wiping from back to front in side-to-side motions, away from the HEPA filter. The solution you should use is isopropyl alcohol (at least 70%).

33. b. Approximately 2 ml per minute. Setup: 500 ml/240 min = x ml/1min; x = 2.08 ml/minute

34. b. An IVPB should run for 30 to 60 minutes. This is not always the case, as there are specific medications that require a longer infusion, but for most mediations this is the standard.

35. b. Each cassette should have a 24-hour supply of medicine in it. Cart exchange of cassettes generally takes place every 24 hours at the same time each day.

36. c. The *United States Pharmacopeia* chapter 797 discusses new and special guidelines not only for making sterile products, but also for preparing or compounding drugs in general.

37. c. A vertical (or chemo) hood is used in the preparation of chemo or cancer drugs or drugs derived from human blood. The vertical hood is more enclosed, not only to help prevent contamination, but also to help prevent the person preparing them from being exposed to the drugs.

38. b. Personal protective equipment is essential when working on hazardous drugs or working in a clean room. These involve a mask, gloves, gown, head cover, and shoe covers, etc.

39. d. They all have the same diameter of 25 G. The volume of the syringe is different, and the length of needle is different in all of them.

40. d. At least 30 minutes. Also, note that the inspection of a laminar flow hood should take place every six months.

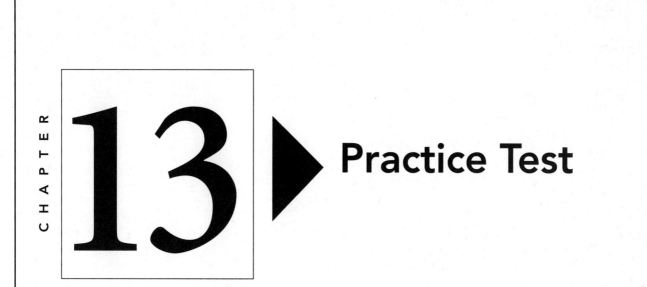

13 ▶ Practice Test

This practice exam is designed to help you prepare for the Pharmacy Technician Exam. It includes the types of questions you are most likely to see on test day. The format is similar to the actual exam as well, so you'll know just what to expect.

In addition to prep for test day, this practice exam is designed to help you identify your strengths and weaknesses. Make a note of the types of questions you miss, and the topics on which you need to further concentrate your study time. Good luck!

1.	(a)	(b)	(c)	(d)
2.	(a)	(b)	(c)	(d)
3.	(a)	(b)	(c)	(d)
4.	(a)	(b)	(c)	(d)
5.	(a)	(b)	(c)	(d)
6.	(a)	(b)	(c)	(d)
7.	(a)	(b)	(c)	(d)
8.	(a)	(b)	(c)	(d)
9.	(a)	(b)	(c)	(d)
10.	(a)	(b)	(c)	(d)
11.	(a)	(b)	(c)	(d)
12.	(a)	(b)	(c)	(d)
13.	(a)	(b)	(c)	(d)
14.	(a)	(b)	(c)	(d)
15.	(a)	(b)	(c)	(d)
16.	(a)	(b)	(c)	(d)
17.	(a)	(b)	(c)	(d)
18.	(a)	(b)	(c)	(d)
19.	(a)	(b)	(c)	(d)
20.	(a)	(b)	(c)	(d)
21.	(a)	(b)	(c)	(d)
22.	(a)	(b)	(c)	(d)
23.	(a)	(b)	(c)	(d)
24.	(a)	(b)	(c)	(d)
25.	(a)	(b)	(c)	(d)
26.	(a)	(b)	(c)	(d)
27.	(a)	(b)	(c)	(d)
28.	(a)	(b)	(c)	(d)
29.	(a)	(b)	(c)	(d)
30.	(a)	(b)	(c)	(d)

31.	(a)	(b)	(c)	(d)
32.	(a)	(b)	(c)	(d)
33.	(a)	(b)	(c)	(d)
34.	(a)	(b)	(c)	(d)
35.	(a)	(b)	(c)	(d)
36.	(a)	(b)	(c)	(d)
37.	(a)	(b)	(c)	(d)
38.	(a)	(b)	(c)	(d)
39.	(a)	(b)	(c)	(d)
40.	(a)	(b)	(c)	(d)
41.	(a)	(b)	(c)	(d)
42.	(a)	(b)	(c)	(d)
43.	(a)	(b)	(c)	(d)
44.	(a)	(b)	(c)	(d)
45.	(a)	(b)	(c)	(d)
46.	(a)	(b)	(c)	(d)
47.	(a)	(b)	(c)	(d)
48.	(a)	(b)	(c)	(d)
49.	(a)	(b)	(c)	(d)
50.	(a)	(b)	(c)	(d)
51.	(a)	(b)	(c)	(d)
52.	(a)	(b)	(c)	(d)
53.	(a)	(b)	(c)	(d)
54.	(a)	(b)	(c)	(d)
55.	(a)	(b)	(c)	(d)
56.	(a)	(b)	(c)	(d)
57.	(a)	(b)	(c)	(d)
58.	(a)	(b)	(c)	(d)
59.	(a)	(b)	(c)	(d)
60.	(a)	(b)	(c)	(d)

61.	(a)	(b)	(c)	(d)
62.	(a)	(b)	(c)	(d)
63.	(a)	(b)	(c)	(d)
64.	(a)	(b)	(c)	(d)
65.	(a)	(b)	(c)	(d)
66.	(a)	(b)	(c)	(d)
67.	(a)	(b)	(c)	(d)
68.	(a)	(b)	(c)	(d)
69.	(a)	(b)	(c)	(d)
70.	(a)	(b)	(c)	(d)
71.	(a)	(b)	(c)	(d)
72.	(a)	(b)	(c)	(d)
73.	(a)	(b)	(c)	(d)
74.	(a)	(b)	(c)	(d)
75.	(a)	(b)	(c)	(d)
76.	(a)	(b)	(c)	(d)
77.	(a)	(b)	(c)	(d)
78.	(a)	(b)	(c)	(d)
79.	(a)	(b)	(c)	(d)
80.	(a)	(b)	(c)	(d)
81.	(a)	(b)	(c)	(d)
82.	(a)	(b)	(c)	(d)
83.	(a)	(b)	(c)	(d)
84.	(a)	(b)	(c)	(d)
85.	(a)	(b)	(c)	(d)
86.	(a)	(b)	(c)	(d)
87.	(a)	(b)	(c)	(d)
88.	(a)	(b)	(c)	(d)
89.	(a)	(b)	(c)	(d)
90.	(a)	(b)	(c)	(d)

This test is similar in format to the PTCB national exam, which you will be given 110 minutes to complete.

1. Which of the following is the most common cleaning agent used within a pharmacy and on a laminar flow hood?
   a. isopropyl alcohol 70%
   b. bleach
   c. soft scrub
   d. dish soap

2. Which of the following describes a formulary drug?
   a. a limited list of drugs found in the pharmacy setting
   b. a list of different formulations of drugs
   c. drugs that are extended- or sustained-release
   d. a compounding principle involving forms of gelatin capsules

3. Which of the following statements is false when talking about a TPN?
   a. It's also known as hyperalimentation.
   b. It's intended for individuals who cannot take anything by mouth.
   c. It's an IV admixture with multiple ingredients, including glucose and protein.
   d. It's administered by mouth, so aseptic technique is not a concern.

4. Which of the following terms is used to define a medication that kills or stops the growth of bacteria in the body?
   a. ACE inhibitor
   b. anticonvulsant
   c. antibiotic
   d. antifungal

5. Which route of administration is used to inject medication into the fatty tissue?
   a. subcutaneous
   b. intramuscular
   c. intravenous
   d. otic

6. The NDC number consists of three sets of digits. What does the first set indicate?
   a. the manufacturer
   b. the product itself
   c. the classification of the drug
   d. the package size

7. A unit dose medication is which of the following?
   a. a medication that has numbers imprinted on it
   b. an individual prepackaged medication
   c. medication used in specific nursing units
   d. a drug that is neither a tablet nor a capsule

8. Of the following drugs, which one is classified as a COX-2 inhibitor?
   a. nifedipine
   b. atenolol
   c. celecoxib
   d. metformin

9. The medication levothyroxine is oftentimes measured in grains. How many milligrams would equal $\frac{1}{200}$ gr?
   a. 0.1 mg
   b. 0.15 mg
   c. 0.2 mg
   d. 0.3 mg

10. What does the abbreviation DUR mean, and which act created this term?

a. drug utilization review; Poison Prevention Packaging Act (PPPA)

b. drug utilization review; FD&C Act

c. drug utilization review; OBRA

d. drug utilization review; Orphan Drug Act

11. The selling price of a drug is $43.29 with a 33% markup and a $7.50 dispensing fee. What is the final cost of this drug?

a. $48.50

b. $54.87

c. $65.08

d. $71.24

12. Of the following needles, which one has the smallest bore, or diameter?

a. 1 ml 27 G$\frac{1}{2}$"

b. 3 ml 23 G1"

c. 5 ml 21 G1"

d. 10 ml 30 G$\frac{3}{4}$"

13. Which of the following routes of administration would bypass the digestive system?

a. oral

b. nasal

c. NG

d. IM

14. Which of the following is a liquid dosage form where the medication is completely dissolved in the solvent?

a. suspension

b. solution

c. emulsion

d. syrup

15. Which of the following is the proper expiration date that should be used when typing a prescription?

a. one year from the date filled

b. two years from the date filled

c. 30 days from the date filled

d. the date indicated on the stock bottle

16. Of the following DEA numbers, which one is correct for Dr. Norma Grimaud?

a. AN 4621858

b. AG 4621853

c. BN 4621852

d. BG 4621858

17. How frequently should a laminar flow hood be serviced?

a. every two months

b. every three months

c. every six months

d. once a year

18. Of the following drugs, which one would be considered a schedule III drug according to the Controlled Substances Act?

a. Percocet®

b. Vicodin®

c. Ambien®

d. Robitussin® with codeine

19. For how many milliliters per minute would one set the administration pump for the following IV admixture?

D51/2NS 1,000 ml to be infused over eight hours

a. approximately 1 ml/min

b. approximately 2 ml/min

c. approximately 3 ml/min

d. approximately 4 ml/min

20. Of the following drugs, which one would be used in the treatment of hypertension?
  a. Singulair®
  b. Depakote®
  c. Tenormin®
  d. Cymbalta®

21. How many milliliters would the following add up to?

0.6 L + 60 ml + 1.5 oz

  a. 690 ml
  b. 705 ml
  c. 755 ml
  d. 545 ml

22. Which of the following is the proper way to clean a laminar flow hood?
  a. back to front of the hood away from the HEPA filter, using side-to-side motions
  b. front to back of the hood toward the HEPA filter, using side-to-side motions
  c. it does not matter as long as you use the correct cleaning agent
  d. up and down, side-to-side, away from the HEPA filter

23. In most hospitals, cart exchange of patient cassettes occurs every
  a. 6 hours.
  b. 12 hours.
  c. 18 hours.
  d. 24 hours.

24. How many milliliters are needed to give an individual dose of 400 mg of the following drug?

FeSO4 220 mg/5 ml 473 ml

  a. 2.2 ml
  b. 4.7 ml
  c. 9.1 ml
  d. 12.4 ml

25. A patient has a question about his or her medication's potential side effects. What should the pharmacy technician do?
  a. inform the patient of potential side effects
  b. give the patient a drug manufacturer's insert, which will have side effects in it
  c. inform the patient not to worry
  d. have the patient see the pharmacist for a consultation

26. The use of aseptic technique involves which of the following?
  a. wearing a new pair of shoes
  b. cleaning the equipment before and after compounding
  c. preparing a sterile product without contaminating it
  d. keeping customers 50 feet from the compounding area

27. How much of a 1:1,000 stock solution is needed to make 360 ml of a 1:2,400 solution?
  a. 10 ml
  b. 100 ml
  c. 150 ml
  d. 240 ml

28. How many milliliters of NPH insulin U-100 will you need to add to the following IV?

D5W 1,000 ml
Add: NPH U-100 35 units

  a. 3.5 ml
  b. 35 ml
  c. 0.35 ml
  d. 350 ml

29. How many grams of NaCl are there in the following IV?

NS 500 ml

a. 0.45 g
b. 4.5 g
c. 0.9 g
d. 9 g

30. The use of safety caps on prescription vials and bottles was mandated by which of the following?

a. OBRA
b. FDA
c. DEA
d. PPPA

31. In which classification of drug would you find Vasotec®?

a. beta-blocker
b. calcium channel blocker
c. ACE inhibitor
d. 5A phosphodiesterase inhibitor

32. Which laminar flow hood should be used when making chemo drugs?

a. horizontal laminar flow hood
b. parallel laminar flow hood
c. vertical laminar flow hood
d. perpendicular laminar flow hood

33. What packaging method does an institutional setting most commonly use?

a. bulk supply
b. unit dose
c. monthly supply
d. individual dose

34. Of the following references, which one has to do with generic equivalencies?

a. *Facts and Comparisons*
b. *OBRA Handbook*
c. *The Orange Book*
d. *Redbook*

35. Which drug formulation would mask the taste of a drug?

a. chewable tablet
b. buccal tablet
c. troche
d. gelatin capsule

36. Licensing or registration of pharmacy technicians is generally done by

a. FDA.
b. DEA.
c. BOP.
d. OBRA.

37. Which of the following was established to set forth compounding standards within pharmacies?

a. USP
b. UPS
c. FDA
d. DEA

38. The dose of drug A is 5 mg/kg body weight. What would the individual dose be for a man who weighs 234 lb?

a. 532 mg
b. 724 mg
c. 850 mg
d. 1,170 mg

39. How many prednisone 5 mg tablets would you dispense for the following directions?

Sig: 40 mg po bid × 2d, 20 mg po qd × 2d, 10 mg po qd × 2d, 5 mg po qd × 2d then dc

a. 24 tablets
b. 32 tablets
c. 46 tablets
d. 60 tablets

40. If you compound a large amount of cream for multiple prescription fills, it would be called
a. extemporaneous compounding.
b. multiple prescription compounding.
c. bulk compounding.
d. a lot of work.

41. 345 oz is equal to how many liters?
a. 3.45 L
b. 7.12 L
c. 10.35 L
d. 12.4 L

42. How much hydrocortisone powder would be found in 4 oz of a 2.5% cream?
a. 3,000 mg
b. 4,000 mg
c. 5,000 mg
d. 6,000 mg

43. Which drops would you use for the following prescription?

Cortisporin® drops 10 ml
Sig: ii gtts au bid × 10d

a. Cortisporin® topical drops
b. Cortisporin® opthalmic drops
c. Cortisporin® otic drops
d. Cortisporin® nasal drops

44. Which medication would be used due to its extended-release formulation?
a. Tylenol Extra Strength®
b. Robitussin DM®
c. Entex LA®
d. Ecotrin EC®

45. D5NS stands for which of the following?
a. dextrose 5% in sterile water
b. dextrose 5% in 0.22% NaCl
c. dextrose 5% in 0.45% NaCl
d. dextrose 5% in 0.9% NaCl

46. You need to measure 48 ml of liquid. What size graduated cylinder would you use?
a. 1 oz
b. 2 oz
c. 3 oz
d. 4 oz

47. The enzyme HMG CoA reductase is involved in synthesizing cholesterol from fat. Which of the following drugs is considered to be an HMG CoA reductase inhibitor?
a. cholestyramine
b. clofibrate
c. pravastatin
d. probucol

48. In the community pharmacy setting, there must be a refrigerator for storing medications that require a storage temperature between
a. 0–4 degrees Celsius.
b. 1–6 degrees Celsius.
c. 2–8 degrees Celsius.
d. 4–10 degrees Celsius.

49. Which of the following is required by regulatory agencies in the pharmacy setting?
- **a.** OSHA guidelines
- **b.** policy and procedures manual
- **c.** *Facts and Comparisons*
- **d.** laminar flow hood

50. One requirement of recertification for either of the national certifying organizations is that the pharmacy technician must participate in continuing education every two years for which of the following lengths of time?
- **a.** 10 contact hours
- **b.** 20 contact hours
- **c.** 30 contact hours
- **d.** 40 contact hours

51. A drug class likely to cause serious adverse reactions or death would be which of the following?
- **a.** class I
- **b.** class II
- **c.** class III
- **d.** class IV

52. The reference book that contains drug manufacturer drug inserts would be which one?
- **a.** *Facts and Comparisons*
- **b.** *OBRA Handbook*
- **c.** *PDR*
- **d.** *The Orange Book*

53. A vial that medication is placed in is measured in
- **a.** milliliters.
- **b.** ounces.
- **c.** drams.
- **d.** scruples.

54. If a patient is on the drug Glucophage®, what is this patient most likely being treated for?
- **a.** hypertension
- **b.** diabetes
- **c.** depression
- **d.** gingival hyperplasia

55. How much of D20W 1,000 ml and D5W 1,000 ml is needed to make D7.5W 500 ml?
- **a.** 83.3 ml D20W and 416.7 ml D5W
- **b.** 416.7 ml D20W and 83.3 ml D5W
- **c.** 102 ml D20W and 398 ml D5W
- **d.** 398 ml D20W and 102 ml D5W

56. For the following IV, what would the infusion rate be in gtts/min?

D51/2NS 1,000 ml over 16 hours
Drop factor: 13 gtts/ml

- **a.** 12 gtts/min
- **b.** 14 gtts/min
- **c.** 16 gtts/min
- **d.** 18 gtts/min

57. How much diluent do you need to add to a 4 g vial to get a concentration of 500 mg/ml? (Note: Disregard the space the powder occupies.)
- **a.** 6 ml
- **b.** 8 ml
- **c.** 10 ml
- **d.** 12 ml

58. The cost of two ounces of triamcinolone acetonide 0.125% is $14.75. What would the cost be for 15 g?
- **a.** $1.20
- **b.** $2.69
- **c.** $3.69
- **d.** $4.19

59. What is the standard flow rate for an IVPB?
  a. 10 to 20 minutes
  b. 30 to 60 minutes
  c. 60 to 90 minutes
  d. 120 minutes

60. Which auxiliary label would you use for the following sig?

  I - ii gtts ad ud prn

  a. take with meals
  b. for the eye
  c. avoid sunlight
  d. for the ear

61. You receive an order for Drug A 12 mg/kg. The patient is four foot seven inches tall and weighs 108 lb. If Drug A comes in a concentration of 250 mg/5 ml 473 ml, how many milliliters would you give the patient for an individual dose?
  a. approximately 8 ml
  b. approximately 12 ml
  c. approximately 14 ml
  d. approximately 16 ml

62. Which of the following medications is used in patients with thyroid hormone deficiency?
  a. Singulair®
  b. Synthroid®
  c. Plavix®
  d. Premarin®

63. Which of the following medications is used for insomnia?
  a. Xanax®
  b. metformin
  c. Ambien®
  d. atenolol

64. You have 1,000 ml of a 70% solution of dextrose. How many kilograms of dextrose are in 200 ml of this solution?
  a. 140 kg
  b. 0.14 kg
  c. 2.8 kg
  d. 0.28 kg

65. Which of the following medications is used for depression?
  a. Prozac®
  b. Flonase®
  c. Altace®
  d. Vicodin®

66. Of the pharmacy reference sources used in the retail pharmacy setting, which one is considered to be the most frequently updated?
  a. *Facts and Comparisons*
  b. *OBRA Handbook*
  c. *PDR*
  d. *The Orange Book*

67. Which of the following medications is used to treat GERD?
  a. nifedipine
  b. trazodone
  c. esomeprazole
  d. enalapril

68. A solution containing 150 mg of drug in 1,000 ml solution would be expressed as which percent?
  a. 0.015%
  b. 0.15%
  c. 1.5%
  d. 15%

69. Using the formula below, what would the temperature in Celsius be if the temperature is 78 degrees Fahrenheit?

$$°C = \frac{(°F - 32)}{1.8}$$

    a. 12.2 degrees
    b. 16.4 degrees
    c. 25.6 degrees
    d. 34.8 degrees

70. How do ACE inhibitors work?
    a. preventing the attachment of angiotensin 2 from attaching to receptor sites
    b. blocking angiotensin receptor sites of the heart
    c. preventing the conversion of angiotensin 1 to angiotensin 2
    d. preventing the stimulation of alpha-2 receptor sites

71. If the expiration date on a prescription reads 12/2010, what is the exact expiration date of this drug?
    a. 11/30/2010
    b. 12/01/2010
    c. 12/31/2010
    d. 1/01/2011

72. A prescription orders 300 milligrams of carbamazepine, but only 200 milligram tablets are available. How many tablets will you dispense?
    a. 2.5
    b. 1.5
    c. 1
    d. 4

73. What is the maximum number of refills allowed for a prescription for zolpidem?
    a. no refills allowed
    b. 3 refills
    c. 5 refills
    d. 11 refills

74. A prescription orders 2.5 grams of neomycin sulfate. 500 milligram tablets are available. How many tablets will you dispense?
    a. two
    b. four
    c. three
    d. five

75. A physician special orders 4 oz of 1.5% betamethasone cream. The pharmacy stocks 2.5% and 1% betamethasone creams. How much of each stock item will a technician need to prepare this compound correctly?
    a. 80 g of 1% and 40 g of 2.5%
    b. 60 g of each strength
    c. 40 g of 1% and 80 g of 2.5%
    d. 90 g of 1% and 30 g of 2.5%

76. The following prescription is brought to the pharmacy: "amoxil liquid 400 mg po tid × 14 days." The pharmacy stocks 500 mg/5 ml amoxicillin suspension. What is the volume of medication needed to fill the entire prescription?
    a. 60 ml
    b. 168 ml
    c. 240 ml
    d. 30 ml

77. What does NaCl mean?
 a. potassium chloride
 b. sodium chloride
 c. calcium chloride
 d. magnesium chloride

78. When a federal law and a state law both exist covering the same issue, which one should be followed?
 a. state law, as this is relevant in the state where you live
 b. federal law, as this supersedes state law
 c. the less stringent of both laws
 d. the more stringent of both laws

79. When storing an item at room temperature, the room should be
 a. 36 to 46 degrees Fahrenheit.
 b. greater than 30 degrees Celsius.
 c. 2 to 8 degrees Celsius.
 d. 15 to 30 degrees Celsius.

80. How many 1 L bags will be needed if D5W is to run 80 ml/hr for 24 hours?
 a. one bag
 b. two bags
 c. three bags
 d. four or more bags

81. What volume of albuterol 5% solution will be needed if 120 ml of 0.05% solution must be compounded for patient use?
 a. 8.3 ml
 b. 0.83 ml
 c. 12 ml
 d. 1.2 ml

82. Of the following medications, which one would be exempt from the Poison Prevention Packaging Act?
 a. clotrimazole troches
 b. verapamil tablets
 c. Nitrostat® SL tablets
 d. ketorolac tablets

83. If a pharmacy wanted to make a 30% profit on an item that was $5.75, what would the retail price need to be?
 a. $1.72
 b. $1.73
 c. $7.48
 d. $2.25

84. How many teaspoons are in a tablespoon?
 a. 2
 b. 3
 c. 4
 d. 5

85. How many tablets are needed if a patient is taking a medication with the directions "1 tab po bid × 7 days"?
 a. 14
 b. 20
 c. 30
 d. 40

86. If a cart exchange is not until 10 A.M. the next day, how many doses should be sent to fill a new patient order received at 2 P.M. for the following medication?

Lopressor® 100 mg po q8h (8 A.M., 4 P.M. and 12 A.M.)

 a. one dose
 b. two doses
 c. three doses
 d. four doses

87. Cyclobenzaprine is a skeletal muscle relaxant. What is its trade or brand name?
   a. Norvasc®
   b. Tenormin®
   c. Flexeril®
   d. Augmentin®

88. The study of absorption, distribution, metabolism, and excretion of a drug in the body is important for giving an exact dose to a patient. This is often referred to as
   a. pharmacognosy.
   b. pharmacology.
   c. pharmacokinetics.
   d. pharmacodynamics.

89. From the following prescription order, how many capsules should you dispense?

Amoxil® 500 mg i po qid × 7d

   a. XXIV
   b. XXVIII
   c. XVIII
   d. XXIX

90. Of the following which information would not be on a unit dose label?
   a. manufacturer
   b. expiration date
   c. patient's name
   d. lot number

Answers and Explanations

1. a. The cleaning agent of choice is isopropyl alcohol, at least 70%. In some cases, bleach such as Clorox® or sodium hypochlorite 10% is used as an alternative.

2. a. A formulary is used in the pharmacy setting mainly because a pharmacy cannot carry all the drugs available, and also due to the cost-effectiveness of using a less expensive drug that will perform the same function as the more expensive one. Insurance companies have their own drug formulary as well.

3. d. Total parenteral nutrition is an IV given to patients who cannot take anything by mouth. TPN contains all that is necessary for nourishment. TPNs are also known as hyperalimentations.

4. c. Antibiotics stop or kill bacteria. ACE inhibitors are for hypertension, anticonvulsants prevent seizures, and antifungals are used for fungal infections.

5. a. Subcutaneous injections penetrate the fatty tissue beneath the skin or dermis. Intramuscular injections penetrate muscle. Intravenous injections put fluid into a vein. And otic simply means "for the ear."

6. a. The NDC number is required on all legend drugs to identify what is inside the container. The first set of digits indicates who the manufacturer is, the second set identifies the drug product itself, and the third set indicates the package size.

7. b. Unit dose medications are used in institutional or hospital pharmacy settings. They are prepackaged units of an individual drug, produced by the drug manufacturer or the pharmacy itself.

8. c. Celecoxib is the same as Celebrex®, a COX-2 inhibitor or antagonist. Nifedipine is a calcium channel blocker, atenolol a beta-blocker, and metformin is what we call a biguanide used for type 2 diabetes.

9. d. To solve this, you simply need to know the ten conversions presented in this review manual. In this case, 1 gr or grain is equal to 60 mg. Set up using ratio and proportion: gr $\frac{1}{60}$ mg = gr $1/400/x$ mg; $x = 0.3$ mg.

10. c. The Drug Utilization Act is part of OBRA, which instructs the pharmacist to do reviews of medications dispensed to a particular patient and ensure there are no mistakes—or if a mistake is found, to correct that mistake. Also part of OBRA is the requirement for pharmacists to counsel patients.

11. c. Selling price = AWP or cost (+ markup or – markdown) – dispensing fee. In this case, the setup would be: $43.29 + $14.29 + $7.50 = $65.08.

12. d. The gauge of a needle indicates the diameter of the needle and its bore (the opening of the needle). The higher the number, the smaller the diameter and bore. In this case, the needle is 30 G, which is higher than the other needle gauges presented.

13. d. Intramuscular administration will bypass the digestive system entirely, while all or part of the other routes will eventually pass through the digestive system.

14. b. Solutions are a liquid dosage form that has the medication completely dissolved in the solvent (liquid). Suspensions and the other formulations presented do not have complete dissolution.

15. d. Always use the date indicated on the stock bottle.

16. d. The first letter of the DEA number is either A or B; the second letter is the first letter of the physician's last name. In calculating whether the number is correct or not, you start by adding the first, third, and fifth numbers to get a total, then add the second, fourth, and sixth numbers (multiplied by 2) to get a second total. Then, you add the two totals—and the last digit of your new number will be the last digit of the DEA number.

17. c. The laminar flow hood should be inspected and serviced, if necessary, every six months.

18. b. Vicodin® is a CIII drug, while Percocet® is CII, Ambien® is CIV, and Robitussin® with codeine is CV.

19. b. Use ratio and proportion. Setup: 1,000 ml/480 ml = x ml/1 min; x = 2.08 ml/min.

20. c. Tenormin®, or atenolol, is a beta-blocker and would be used in the treatment of hypertension. Singulair® is for allergies, Depakote® for seizure control, and Cymbalta® for depression.

21. b. Setup: 600 ml + 60 ml + 45 ml = 705 ml.

22. a. The correct way to clean the laminar flow hood is from top to bottom on the sides, then back to front, using side-to-side motions away from the HEPA filter. Isopropyl alcohol 70% should be used.

23. d. Cart exchange for cassette drawers occurs once a day, or every 24 hours. That is why it is important to have a 24-hour supply of unit dose medication in each cassette drawer.

24. c. Use ratio and proportion. Setup: 220 mg/5 ml = 400 mg/x ml; x = 9.09 ml.

25. d. Any question or concern from a customer or patient that requires an educational judgmental decision should be given to the pharmacist to address. This would include counseling.

26. c. Aseptic technique is the preparation of a sterile product without contaminating it. The other answers may be examples, but are not the true definition.

27. c. Use ratio and proportion. First, find out how many grams you need from your product. Setup: 1 g/2,400 ml = x g/360 ml, x = 0.15 g. The new setup would be: 1 g/1,000 ml = 0.15 g/x ml; x = 150 ml.

28. c. To solve this, you need to know that the standard for insulin is 1 ml – 100 units. Use ratio and proportion. Setup: 1 ml/100 units = x ml/35 units; x = 0.35 ml.

29. b. To solve this you need to know that NS is normal saline, which is the same as 0.9% NaCl. Use ratio and proportion. Setup: 0.9 g/100 ml = x g/500 ml; x = 4.5 g.

30. d. The use of safety caps for all prescriptions that leave the pharmacy was mandated by the Poison Prevention Packaging Act.

31. c. Vasotec® or enalapril is what we call an ACE inhibitor or angiotensin converting enzyme inhibitor. Looking at the ending of the generic name of these drugs (-*pril*) helps you to know what its classification is.

32. c. The vertical, or chemo, hood is used in preparing hazardous materials such as chemo drugs used for cancer patients. The horizontal hood is for preparing sterile products. In this question, the other hoods listed as answer choices do not exist.

33. b. Unit dose is the most commonly used dosing method in the institutional/hospital setting. One thing to note about unit doses is that if the medication is not opened, it can be reused.

34. c. *The Orange Book* contains information on the bioequivalencies of generic drugs. *Facts and Comparisons* is the most widely used reference source on drugs used in the pharmacy setting. The *Redbook* deals with the AWP of prescription drugs.

35. d. The gelatin capsule is used to hold medication, thus masking the taste of drugs as well as allowing a formulation that is easier to swallow. Sometimes drug manufacturers will place a whole tablet into a capsule, which is known as "bulleting."

36. c. The state board of pharmacy is involved in the licensing and registration of not only pharmacy technicians, but pharmacists and pharmacies as well.

37. a. The *United States Pharmacopeia* (USP) sets standards for drugs, ensuring a safe product.

38. a. Use ratio and proportion. Setup: 5 mg/2.2 lb = x mg/234 lb; x = 531.82 mg.

39. c. 40 mg, or eight tabs twice a day for two days, is equal to 32 tabs. 20 mg, or four tabs once a day for two days, is equal to eight tabs. 10 mg, or two tabs once a day for two days, is equal to four tabs. Finally, 5 mg, or one tab daily for two days, is two tabs. The total would be 32 + 8 + 4 + 2 = 46 tabs.

40. c. Compounding multiple prescriptions is called bulk compounding. Compounding for one prescription order only is called extemporaneous compounding. There is no reason why a pharmacy technician cannot legally compound.

41. c. Use ratio and proportion. Setup: 1 L/1,000 ml = x L/10,350 ml; x = 10.35 L.

42. a. Use ratio and proportion. Setup: 2,500 mg/100 g = x mg/120 g; x = 3,000 mg.

43. c. Cortisporin® otic drops indicate two drops into each ear. Cortisporin® ophthalmic drops would be used for the eye.

44. c. LA indicates that the drug is long-acting. DM indicates the other drug included, which is dextromethorphan. EC means the drug is enteric-coated to bypass the stomach.

45. d. D5NS is dextrose 5% in normal saline, which is the same as 0.9% NaCl.

46. b. When measuring accurately, try to use the next larger-sized container, whether this involves a bottle, vial, graduate, or syringe. In this case, you would use a 2 oz, or 60 ml, container to measure 48 ml. You can use the 3 oz or 4 oz container, but it would not be as accurate.

47. c. Pravastatin, or Pravachol®, is an HMG-CoA redutase inhibitor or antagonist. The ending of the generic name, -*statin*, tells you the classification of this drug.

48. c. In the pharmacy setting, Celsius is the temperature standard. For drugs requiring refrigeration, the temperature should be between 2 to 8 degrees Celsius.

49. b. The policy and procedures manual, which contains protocols for most situations that may arise in the pharmacy setting, is required.

50. b. For both national certification organizations, you are required to complete 20 hours minimum of continuing education every two years—one hour of which must be in pharmacy law.

51. a. There are three drug recalls with class 1, in which a serious adverse reaction is possible, being the most serious. Class II is less serious, and class III means that the product does not meet FDA guidelines.

52. c. *PDR* is more of a marketing tool for drug companies, as it contains only drug inserts and information that drug manufacturers want in it. The *PDR* also contains information about how to contact drug companies and poison control centers.

53. c. A vial for medication (such as tablets and capsules) is measured in drams. The larger the vial, the greater the dram size. Vials and bottles for liquid formulations are brown or amber in color, due to the possibility of degradation in sunlight.

54. b. Glucophage®, or metformin, is used for type 2 diabetes mellitus.

55. a. Using the allegation chart, you get $(\frac{2.5}{15})(500$ ml) = 83.3 ml of the D20W, and $(\frac{12.5}{15})(500$ ml) = 416.7 ml of D5W.

56. b. Use ratio and proportion. Setup: 1,000 ml/960 min = x ml/1 min; x = 10.4 ml/min. The next step is to multiply this by your drop factor: (10.4 ml/min) (13 gtts/ml) = 13.54 gtts/min, or 14 gtts/min.

57. b. Use ratio and proportion. Setup: 500 mg/ml = 4,000 mg/x ml; x = 8 ml.

58. c. Use ratio and proportion. Setup: $14.75/60 g = x/15 g; x = $3.69.

59. b. The standard flow rate for IVPB is 30 to 60 minutes; however, depending on the medication, this time frame can be longer.

60. d. Because the sig (directions) indicate the drops are to be placed in the right ear, we would use the auxiliary label "for the ear."

61. b. This question involves two-part problem solving using ratio and proportion. Step 1 for dose: 12 mg/2.2 lb = x mg/108 lb; x = 589.09 mg. Step 2 for volume needed: 250 mg/5 ml = 589.09 mg/x ml; x = 11.78 ml.

62. b. Synthroid® treats hormone deficiency. Singulair® treats allergies, Plavix® treats clots, and Premarin® is used to treat menopause.

63. c. Ambien® is used for insomnia. Xanax® is used for anxiety, metformin is used for diabetes, and atenolol is used for hypertension.

64. b. Use ratio and proportion to solve for grams. Setup: 70 g/100 ml = x g/200 ml; x = 140 g. The next setup converts the answer to kilograms: 1 kg/1,000 g = x kg/140 g; x = 0.14 kg.

65. a. Prozac® treats depression. Altace® treats hypertension, Flonase® treats allergies, and Vicodin® treats pain.

66. a. *Facts and Comparisons* comes in a three-ring binder that is updated each month with new drug inserts mailed to the pharmacy to replace old inserts.

67. c. Esomeprazole, or Nexium®, is used to treat GERD (gastroesophageal reflux disease). Nifedipine and enalapril treat hypertension, and trazodone treats depression.

68. a. Use ratio and proportion. Setup: 0.15 g/1,000 ml = x g/100 ml, x = 0.015 g; the definition of 0.015 g/100 ml is 0.015%.

69. c. C = (78 − 32)/1.8 = 25.6 degrees Celsius.

70. c. ACE inhibitors work by preventing the reaction of A1 converting to A2, which causes vasoconstriction that can lead to high blood pressure.

71. c. When the expiration date is written in month and year format, the true expiration date will be the last day of the month and year indicated. In this case, the expiration date is 12/31/2010.

72. b. Use ratio and proportion. Setup: 1 tab/200 mg = x tabs/300 mg. 1.5 tablets of 200 mg carbamazepine will give a 300 mg dose.

73. c. For controlled drugs CIII to CV, the maximum number of refills is 5. Zolpidem, or Ambien®, is a CIV drug. For CII drugs, refills cannot be given; and for noncontrolled drugs, the maximum number of refills allowed is 11.

74. d. Use ratio and proportion. Setup: 1 tab/500 mg = x tabs/2,500 mg; x = 5 tabs.

75. a. Using the allegation chart, you get $\frac{0.5}{1.5} \times 120$ = 40 g of the 2.5%, and $\frac{1}{1.5} \times 120$ = 80 g of 1%.

76. b. 400 mg 3 times a day × 14 days = 16,800 mg. Use ratio and proportion to solve. Setup: 16,800 mg/x ml = 500 mg/5 ml; x = 168 ml.

77. b. Na is sodium and Cl is chlorine, so NaCl is sodium chloride. Another example would be that K (potassium) and Cl (chloride) become KCl, potassium chloride.

78. d. When it comes to following state law versus federal law, legally you should follow the most stringent law.

79. d. 15 to 30 degrees Celsius is 59 to 86 degrees Fahrenheit, which is the correct room temperature.

80. b. Use ratio and proportion. Setup: 80 ml/1 hr = x ml/24 hrs = 1,920 ml = 2 L bags.

81. d. Using the allegation chart, you get $(\frac{0.005}{5})$ (120) = 1.2 ml of the 5% solution.

82. c. The Poison Prevention Packaging Act requires the use of safety caps for all medications that leave the pharmacy, unless a patient requests and signs a waiver not to have one—or specific medication like nitroglycerin, or Nitrostat®, is prescribed. Nitrostat® is the trade name for nitroglycerin (the drug used for the disease state angina), which is used in emergency situations where the patient must be able to take the medication as soon as possible.

83. c. $\frac{\$5.75}{100} = \frac{x}{30}$; 100$x$ = 172.5; x = 1.73; $1.73 + $5.75 = $7.48.

84. b. 5 ml = 1 teaspoon and 15 ml = 1 tablespoon. Setup: 5 ml/1 tsp = 15 ml/x tsp; x = 3 teaspoons.

85. a. Follow the directions and multiply: (1 tablet) (2 per day)(7 days) = 14 tablets.

86. c. You will need to give a dose for 4 P.M., 12 a.m., and 8 A.M., as these doses are before the next cart exchange at 10 A.M.

87. c. Cyclobenzaprine is the same as Flexeril®. Norvasc® is felodipine, Tenormin® is atenolol, and Augmentin® is amoxicillin and clavulanic acid, or clavulinate.

88. c. Pharmacokinetics is used to get as exact a dose as possible for drugs that are in what is called a narrow therapeutic window. Pharmacognosy is the study of medicinal ingredients in plants. Pharmacology is the study of the mechanism of drug action in the body. Pharmacodynamics is the study of the physiological effects a drug has on the body or microorganisms within the body.

89. b. If you decide the Roman numerals, they tell us the correct number of capsules to give is 28.

90. c. A unit dose is an individual, prepackaged unit of medication that will include the name of the drug, strength, manufacturer, lot number, and expiration date on it.

GLOSSARY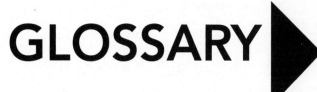

accuracy   the degree of truth of a measurement

adulteration   the tampering or contamination of a product or substance

adverse effect   a harmful or undesired side effect resulting from the use of a medication

aerobic   needing oxygen to survive

allegation   method to find the amount of each ingredient needed to make a mixture of a given quantity or concentration

ampule   a small sealed vial which is used to contain and preserve a drug, usually a liquid commonly made of glass; abbreviated amp

anaerobic   the ability to survive without oxygen

anatomy   the study of the structures of the body

antibiotic   a substance that has the ability to destroy or interfere with the development of a living organism

apothecary   an old English system of weight and volume measures

application software   any software that is used by a facility in the administration of care

Arabic numeral   the ten digits (0, 1, 2, 3, 4, 5, 6, 7, 8, and 9); the standard conventional numbers

arteries   the large vessels that carry oxygen-rich blood

American Association of pharmacy technicians (AAPT)   a nonprofit organization specifically for pharmacy technicians in the offering of CE, information, and networking opportunites with fellow pharmacy technicians nationwide; established 1979

Average Wholesale Price (AWP)   price used by pharmacy in the pricing of prescriptions to third party insurance companies; the AWP can be found in the *Redbook*

bactericidal   an agent that kills microorganisms

bacteriostatic   an agent that inhibits but does not kill microorganisms

blood   a liquid tissue that is responsible for life, growth, and health; it contains red blood cells, white blood cells, and platelets suspended in blood plasma

broad-spectrum antibiotic   a drug that has an antibacterial spectrum against a wide variety of organisms

buccal   located between the gum and the skin of the cheek

capsule   a solid dosage form in which the drug is enclosed within either a hard or soft soluble container or shell usually made of gelatin; abbreviated cap

cardiac muscle   found exclusively in the heart, it is responsible for pumping blood throughout the body

case law   a system of law based on judges' decisions and legal precedents

centi-   the metric system prefix indicating one-hundredth

centigrade   the standard metric system temperature scale of 100 degrees, with 0 being the freezing point and 100 being the boiling point of water

central nervous system   the part of the nervous system that contains the brain and spinal cord; it is responsible for controlling all nervous function

centralized pharmacy   a pharmacy that provides its services from one location

clean room   bacteria-free room used in the preparation of sterile products such as IV admixtures

code of ethics   a set of standards and principles that guide professionals in their functions

common fraction   an expressed number of parts of a whole

common law   a system of law derived from the decision of judges rather than statute

compound   a substance made up of two or more elements

compromised host   a person whose normal defense system is impaired and who is more susceptible to disease

computer applications   the hardware and software utilized to administer healthcare in a specific setting

computer hardware   the physical components of a computer system; includes the mouse, keyboard, and monitor

concentration   measure of how much of a given substance there is mixed with another substance; most frequently limited to homogeneous solutions, where it refers to the amount of solute in the solvent

contract law   a system of law that binds parties to a set of agreements

controlled substances   any medication that has the potential for abuse or dependency liability, as defined by the Controlled Substances Act of 1972

cream   topical preparation usually for application to the skin or to mucus membranes, such as those of the rectum or vagina

criminal law   the body of law that defines criminal offenses against the public

cubic centimeter   a measure of volume equal to a one cube centimeter on a side; often used in the past interchangeably with milliliter; *avoid using this unit because of the possibility of medication error*

daily dose   total amount of drug administered in a 24-hour period

decentralized pharmacy   a pharmacy that has a main location from which it provides services, but also has services in the patient care areas

decimal fraction   a decimal number with a value less than one and greater than zero; there is a zero to the left of the decimal point (e.g., 0.25)

decimal number   a numerator expressed in numerals with a decimal point placed to designate the value of the denominator, which is understood to be ten or a power of ten (100, 1,000, etc.)

delayed-release   formulation used in tablets or capsules to delay release of the drug

denominator   the part of a fraction that is below the fraction bar and that functions as the divisor of the numerator

diluent   agent used to increase the bulk weight or volume of a dosage form

dilution   process of making something less concentrated

direct purchasing   when a pharmacy purchases pharmaceutical supplies directly from the manufacturer

dosage   measured portion of medicine; also called dose

dosage form   the physical form of a dose of medication given for administration (for example, capsule, solution, cream)

dose   the quantity of medication given to a patient as prescribed by a physician

drug class   a group of medications that have the same mechanism of action or chemical properties used to treat a specific disease/diseases

drug classification   a group of medications with the same or similar characteristics

Drug Enforcement Agency (DEA)   a regulatory body that oversees the manufacturing and distribution of controlled substances; tt also focuses on major trafficking of illegal drugs

drug utilization review (DUR)   the process used by the retail pharmacy system to compare the existing treatment to a new treatment's compatibility

drug wholesaler   a third party that purchases medications directly from the manufacturer and sells it to the pharmacy

effervescent   the escape of gas from an aqueous solution

elixir   a sweet flavored liquid usually containing a small amount of alcohol and medication to be taken by mouth in order to mask an unpleasant taste; abbreviated elix

emulsifying agent   a compound that facilitates the formation of an emulsion

emulsion   a suspension of small globules of one liquid in a second liquid with which the first will not mix; an emulsion may be oil-in-water or water-in-oil

endocrine system   a collection of glands that secrete hormones which regulate the body's functions

enema   the introduction of a liquid or foam through the anus used for treatment or diagnosis

enteric-coated (EC)   a barrier applied to oral medications that controls the location in the digestive system where it is absorbed

ethics   the study of values, morals, or morality, including concepts of good and evil, right and wrong

excipient   an inactive substance used as a carrier for the active ingredients of a medication

extended-release   used in pills, tablets, or capsules to dissolve slowly and release a drug over time

extremes the two outside terms in a proportion

Fahrenheit   standard household system temperature scale

film-coated   a barrier applied to oral medication that facilitates swallowing and masks unpleasant tastes

filter needle   a needle that has a filter that will take out anything greater than five microns; used in the removal of ampule contents; also available are filter straws for the same purpose

flow rate   the amount of fluid that flows in a given time

fluid ounce   the measure of volume in the apothecary system equal to 28.57 mL

Food and Drug Administration (FDA)   governmental regulatory agency whose purpose is to ensure safety and efficacy of all drugs currently on the market

formulary   a list of drugs that can be ordered, stocked, and administered at a given facility; also a term used for insurance companies as far as what medications they will pay for

fraction   an expression of division; a number that is a portion or part of a whole (e.g., $\frac{2}{3}$)

fraud   the intentional deceit to deprive another or his or her money, property, or rights

gallon   household measure of volume equal to eight pints

gastrointestinal system   system made up of the stomach and large and small intestines; it is responsible for absorbing nutrients into the body

gel   jelly like material that can have properties ranging from soft and weak to hard and tough

general ledger   the document that keeps a record for all debits and credits of a business

generic name   a general name given to a medication, which is not proprietary

grain   standard unit of weight in the apothecary system; 1 grain (gr) is equal to 64.82 mg

gram   standard unit of weight in the metric system; 1 gram (g) is equal to 1,000 mg

granule   wetted powders allowed to dry and then ground into course pieces having a particle size larger than powders

heart   made of cardiac muscle, this organ is responsible for pumping deoxygenated blood to the lungs and oxygenated blood to the rest of the body

HEPA filter   filtration system used in laminar flow hoods to remove any particles less than 0.2 to 0.3 microns to ensure a steril (bacteria-free) work area

hydro-alcoholic   solvent containing water and alcohol

hydrophilic   anything mixable with water

hypertonic   having an osmotic pressure greater than human plasma; greater than 0.9% NaCl

hypotonic   having an osmotic pressure less than human plasma; less than 0.9% NaCl

improper fraction   a fraction in which the numerator is greater than or equal to the denominator

indication   the intended use of a medication; what it treats

infusion   the introduction of a solution into a vein over a prolonged period of time

inhalation   medication to be taken by drawing in of air (or other gases), as in breathing

inhaler   a device used for inhalation; MDI means metered dose inhaler

injection   a method of putting liquid into the body, usually with a hollow needle and a syringe which is pierced through the skin to a sufficient depth for the material to be forced into the body

integumentary system   also known as the skin, it is responsible for protecting the internal structures from the external environment

international unit   standard amount of a drug required to produce a certain effect

inventory turns   the number of times the entire inventory was purchased over a certain period of time, usually one year

isotonic   term applied to two solutions with equal solute concentrations having the same or equal osmotic pressure; having an osmotic pressure equal to that of human plasma; equal to 0.9% NaCl

jelly   see gel

kilo-   metric system prefix indicating one-thousand

laminar flow hood (LFH)   hood used in the preparation of sterile products such as IV admixtures; two types: horizontal for general preparation and vertical for chemo drugs

law   a rule of conduct or procedure established by custom, agreement, or authority

legal precedent   a legal principle created by a court decision that provides an example for judges deciding similar issues in future cases

legend drug   another name for a prescription drug

legislative law   law that is enacted by legislative decisions; also known as statutory law

liter   standard unit of volume in the metric system; 1 liter (L) is equal to 1,000 milliliters (mL)

lotion   a low- to medium-viscosity, topical preparation intended for application to unbroken skin

lowest common denominator   the smallest whole number that can be divided evenly by all denominators of a series of fractions

lozenge   solid dosage form intended to dissolve or disintegrate slowly in the mouth, usually in a flavored, sweetened base

malpractice   professional misconduct or lack of knowledge which results in injury, death, or damage to a patient

markup   the difference between the cost of an item and the price for which it sells

means   the two inside terms of a proportion

mechanism of action (MOA)   how the medication affects the body or disease to cure or treat a condition

medication error   a broad term that defines the potentially unsafe or unauthorized use of a medication on a patient

medication order   used in the inpatient setting to prescribe medications to a patient

metric system   standard system of measure used throughout most of the world and exclusively in the scientific community; most common system of measure in pharmacy

micro-   metric system prefix indicating one-millionth

milli-   metric system prefix indicating one-thousandth

misbranding   fraudulent or misleading labeling or marketing

misdemeanor   a crime that is punishable by a fine or up to one year in jail

mixed fraction   a combination of a whole number and a proper fraction; the value of a mixed fraction is always greater than one

National Association of the Boards of Pharmacy (NABP)   the professional association that helps to develop uniform standards for all states involved in the practice of pharmacy, with a focus on the protection of public health

net profit   the amount left from the selling price after cost of operations and overhead have been deducted

normal saline   0.9% sodium chloride solution that is isotonic to body fluids; symbolized by NS; 0.9 g NaCl per 100 ml solution

numerator   the expression written above the line in a common fraction and which functions as the dividend of the denominator

ointment   thick viscous preparation for application to the skin, often containing medication; abbreviated ung

ophthalmic   pertaining to the eye

oral   relating to, affecting, or for use in the mouth or administration by way of the mouth

orphan drug   a drug that is used to treat rare diseases, defined by the FDA as fewer than 200,000 people in the United States

otic   pertaining to the ear

ounce   measure of weight in the apothecary system equal to approximately 30 grams (g)

ovaries   the female sex organs responsible for producing estrogen; these also contain the eggs which are released during the menstrual cycle

overhead   the cost of doing business

parenteral   avoiding the gastrointestinal tract

paste   preparation for external application that is usually stiffer, less greasy, and more hydrophilic than ointments

pastilles   subclass of lozenges that are softer and contain a high concentration of sugar or gelatin

pathology   the study of diseases in the body

patient profile   a written or electronic file that contains all of the patient's demographic information

percent   a fraction whose numerator is expressed and whose denominator is understood to be 100; symbolized by %; in pharmacy, a percent is defined as grams of active drug/100 mL solution or g of base

percent markup   markup expressed as a percent of cost

pH   a measure of the relative acidity or alkalinity of a solution or substance

pharmacodynamics   the study of the physiological changes that occur when a medication is introduced into the body

pharmacokinetics   the study of how a medication moves and changes throughout the body

physiology   the study of the functions of the body

pint   household measure of volume equal to 16 fluid ounces

policy   a plan of action that sets limits or boundary conditions around decisions that employees make

powder   intimate mixtures of dry, finely divided drugs and/or inert ingredients intended for internal or external use

preservative   a substance used to retard, minimize, or prevent growth of microorganisms

procedure   a stepwise view of how to execute a specific task

product   the result of multiplying two or more quantities together

professional ethics   standards that guide an individual in their profession

proper fraction   a fraction in which the numerator is smaller than the denominator; the value of a proper fraction is always less than one

proportion   the relationship between two equal ratios

protected health information   any communication that can identify an individual or disclose information about the state of their health; abbreviated as PHI

purchase order (PO)   the document sent to a medication supplier which requests an order of medication be sent to the pharmacy

Pyxis®   a machine that dispenses medication as well as durable medical products; used today in many hospital institutions, pharmacies, and nursing units

quart   a household measure of volume equal to 32 fluid ounces

ratio   an expression that compares two numbers by division; symbolized by a colon

ratio strength   a measure of concentration that specifies a quantity of substance in grams contained in a specified volume of solution; for example, ratio strength of 1:1,000 means 1 g dissolved in 1,000 mL of solution

reconstitution   the preparation of a powder bottle/vial into a liquid formulation by adding necessary diluent (liquid)

rectal   pertaining to the final straight portion of the large intestine

repackaged medications   any pharmacy product that has been removed from its original packaging from the manufacturer and placed in new packaging by the pharmacy

respiratory system   the organ system that contains the lungs, which is responsible for taking in oxygen and excreting carbon dioxide

Roman numeral   the system of numerals that uses letters to represent number values

rounding   a process to yield a new number that has about the same value as the original number, but is less exact

saline   salt solution, usually composed of sodium chloride

selling price   the amount the customer pays for the product or service

solute   any substance that is dissolved in a liquid solvent to create a solution

solution   homogeneous (evenly distributed) mixture of two or more substances, frequently (but not necessarily) a liquid; abbreviated sol

solvent   a liquid substance capable of dissolving other substances

state board of pharmacy (BOP)   the governing body that determines practice standards in a particular state

stock solution   a concentrated solution that is diluted before use

subcutaneous   beneath the skin; abbreviated SQ, SC, or subQ

sublingual   placed beneath the tongue; abbreviated SL

suppository   a small plug of medication designed for insertion into the rectum or vagina where it melts; abbreviated supp

suspension   a mixture in which fine particles are suspended in a fluid where they are supported by buoyancy; abbreviated "susp"

syrup   thick liquid to which a sweetener has been added to mask the taste of a bitter drug or to make it easier for children to take; abbreviated syr

tablespoon   a household measurement of volume approximately equal to 15 mL

tablet   a dose of medicine in the form of a small pellet; abbreviated tab

teaspoon   a household measurement of volume approximately equal to 5 mL

testes   the male sex organs responsible for secreting testosterone; responsible for producing sperm

thyroid gland   endocrine gland that secretes thyroid hormone; responsible for regulating metabolism and generating body heat

tincture   a medicine consisting of an extract in a strong alcohol solution; abbreviated tr

topical   pertaining to the surface of a body part

transdermal   through the skin

troche   subcategory of lozenge that is compressed

unit   the amount of medication required to produce a desired effect

veins   the large vessels that carry oxygen-depleted blood

vial   a relatively small glass vessel used to store medication as liquid or powder

ADDITIONAL ONLINE PRACTICE ▶

Whether you need help building basic skills or preparing for an exam, visit the LearningExpress Practice Center! On this site, you can access additional practice materials. Using the code below, you'll be able to log in and take an additional practice Pharmacy Technician Exam. This online practice will also provide you with:

- **Immediate scoring**
- **Detailed answer explanations**
- **Personalized recommendations for further practice and study**

Log in to the LearningExpress Practice Center by using this URL: **www.learnatest.com/practice**

This is your Access Code: **7373**

Follow the steps online to redeem your access code. After you've used your access code to register with the site, you will be prompted to create a username and password. For easy reference, record them here:

Username: _____   **Password:**_____

With your username and password, you can log in and answer these practice questions as many times as you like. If you have any questions or problems, please contact LearningExpress customer service at 1-800-295-9556 ext. 2, or e-mail us at **customerservice@learningexpressllc.com**.

NOTES

NOTES

NOTES

NOTES

NOTES

NOTES